Four-We Bikini Body

by Joe Warner

Art Editor Ian Ferguson
Photography Simon Howard
Managing Editor Chris Miller
Model Talia Marshall
Additional Photography iStock

Model's clothing supplied by Manduka (manduka.com)
and Under Armour (underarmour.co.uk)

Publisher Steven O'Hara
Publishing Director Dan Savage
Marketing Manager Charlotte Park
Commercial Director Nigel Hole

Printed by William Gibbons and Sons, Wolverhampton

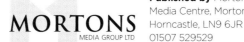

Published by Mortons Media Group Ltd,
Media Centre, Morton Way,
Horncastle, LN9 6JR
01507 529529

To license this product please contact Carlotta Serantoni on +44 (0) 20 79076550 or email carlotta_serantoni@dennis.co.uk
To syndicate content from this product please contact Ryan Chambers on +44(0) 20 7907 6132 or email Ryan_Chambers@dennis.co.uk

Contents

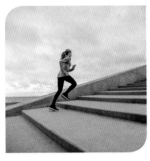
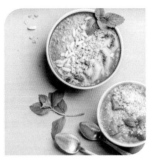
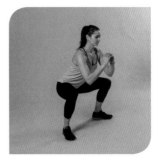
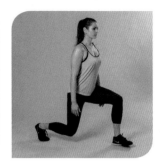
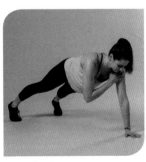
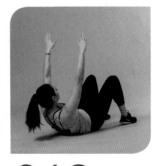
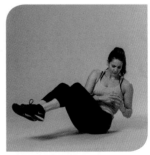
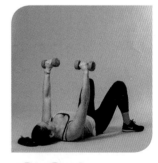

102

WEEKS 1-4
Here's all the workouts
for the advanced plan
to push you harder to
transform your body so you
look and feel fantastic.

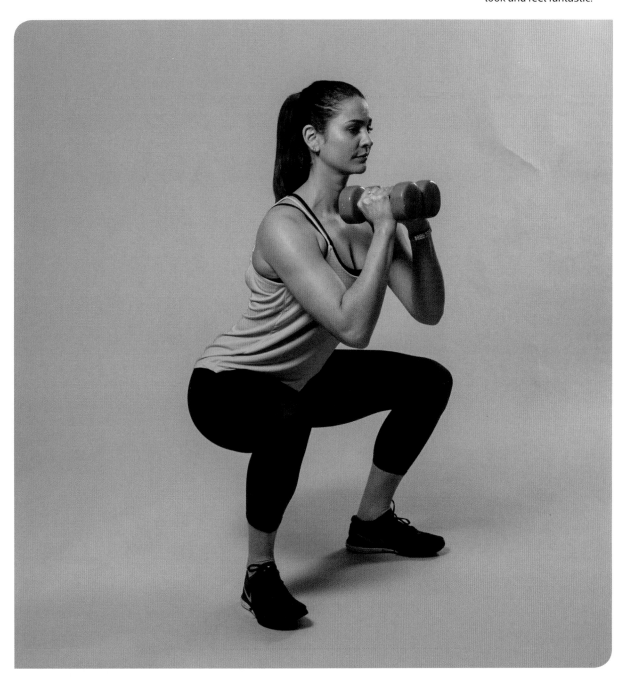

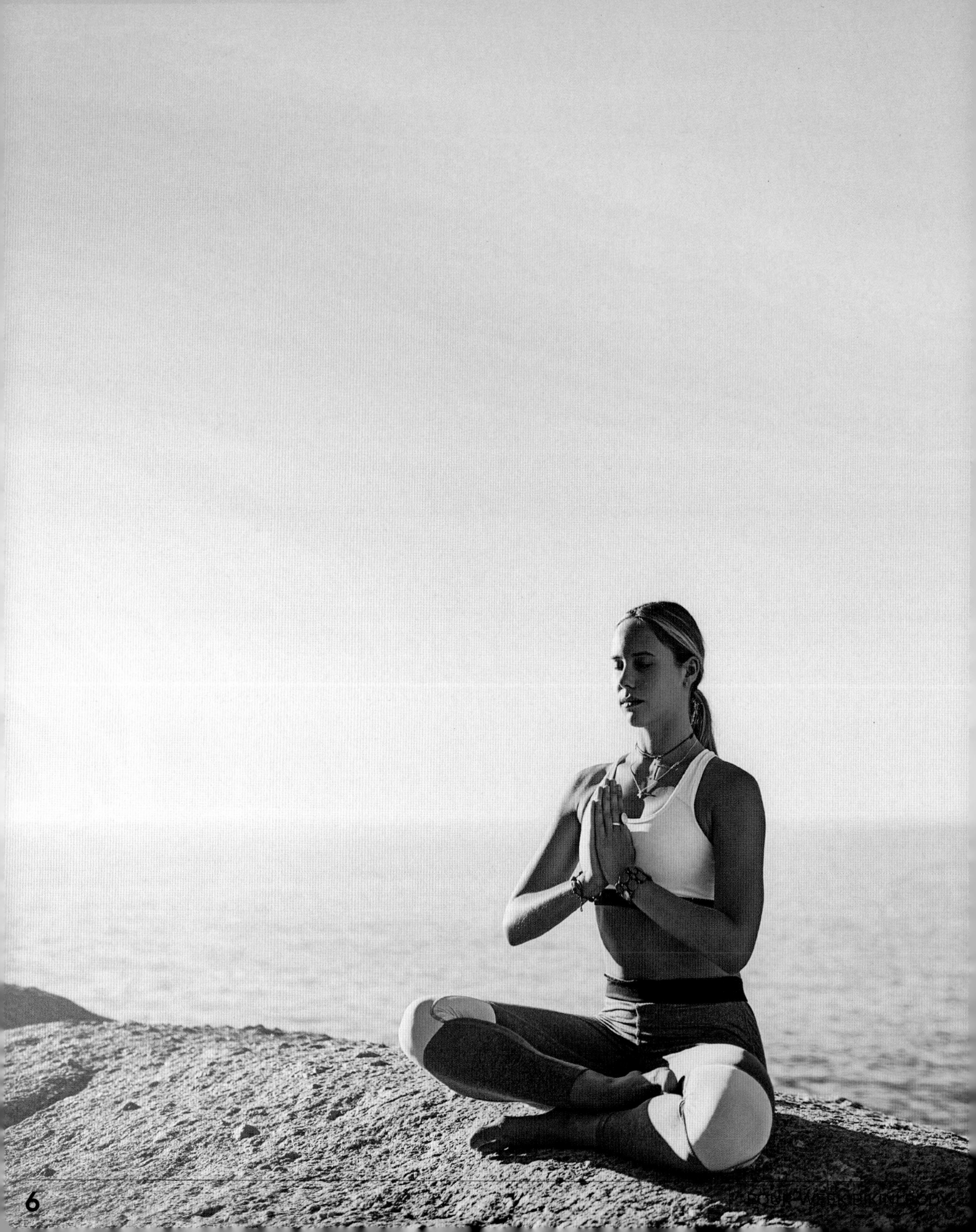

You're four weeks from a bikini body!

Follow our lifestyle advice, eating guide and exercise plan to lose fat and get toned muscles

Welcome to your *Four-Week Bikini Body* exercise and eating guide! Building your best-ever body has never been this easy!

When most people try to lose fat quickly they do one of two things: they either start going for lots of long slow runs; or they drastically cut how many calories they eat each day. Now, both of those approaches will burn body fat for a week, or maybe two at most. But these weight-loss strategies are unsustainable. In the first scenario you quickly run out of energy and motivation to maintain your time-consuming jogging habit, and will likely suffer multiple aches, pains or even injuries. In the second scenario, dropping certain foods or even entire food groups from your diet also means you very quickly feel tired and lethargic, and constantly crave all those foods you're denying yourself. In both instances, it's not surprising that most people then put back on more weight than they've lost once they finally throw in the towel on their new but short-lived exercise or eating plan.

So what is the answer to the question of what's the best way to lose body fat and sculpt a lean and defined body as quickly as possible? To achieve this goal, you need to get smart! And that's exactly what this book is

all about: giving you smart exercise, eating and lifestyle advice so you can lose weight in a simple, sustainable and - most importantly - enjoyable way! In this book you'll find instantly-applicable advice on how to quickly and easily adopt new daily habits that will turn your body into a calorie-burning machine - even when you're not working out! There's also a comprehensive guide on how to eat for a healthier and happier life, without the need to eliminate foods or radically reduce your daily calorie intake.

And then you'll find your *Four-Week Bikini Body* training programme, comprising three sessions per week for a month. If you thought that it was impossible to make big changes to your body in just 12 sessions, be prepared to be amazed by the progress you make when you follow our specially-designed plan to the letter. Then, once you've completed your four-week plan, we've included an advanced month-long plan to take your results to an even more impressive level. This advanced plan uses dumbbells to push your heart and muscles harder so that your body has no choice but to continue burning fat and sculpting stronger and more defined muscles. So read on then put our advice into action and discover the smart yet simple way to exercise and eat to look and feel better than ever!

FAQ

Q
HOW MUCH FAT WILL I LOSE?

Q
WHAT ABOUT CARDIO?

Q
WILL I BE OK TO DO THIS PLAN?

Q
DO I HAVE TO CHANGE MY DIET?

Q
HOW CAN I GET MOTIVATED?

Q
WHAT ELSE SHOULD I DO?

How much body fat you'll lose doing this plan depends on many factors, including: your age; previous training experience; previous weight history; quality and quanity of sleep; how hard you push yourself when training; how well you eat, and more besides. So while it's impossible to estimate how much you'll lose, remember that if you make getting leaner and healthier your priority for the next four weeks then you will make some major progres in how good you look and feel!

Many people think - wrongly - that doing lots of jogging or other types of long cardio is the best way to lose weight. This plan instead focuses on the scientifically-proven smart way to burn body fat fastest: resistance training. Working your body against your own bodyweight - doing squats, lunges and press-ups - not only gets your heart rate high - just like when doing intense cardio - it also breaks down muscle tissue, which your body then rebuilds stronger to make them more defined.

Sometimes it can be a bit scary to start a new exercise plan that is based on an approach you haven't tried before. So if most of the exercise you've done is cardio or other forms of training that's not resistance-based, don't be concerned! The plan starts off using very simple exercises with easy-to-understand movement patterns, and every exercise is demonstrated with both photos and written form guides, so you can do every move effectively and safely to start torching fat.

Increasing your activity levels through a structured exercise plan is one of the most important steps you can take to lose fat and improve your health. But just as important to your overall health and happiness levels is what you eat - not just for one day or one month- but over the long term by following a simple and sustainable approach to food and eating. Starting from p18 you'll discover the smart ways to make some quick and easy changes to your diet that will give your body all the nutrients it needs to thrive.

Ultimately, you are the only person who can determine how much - and how quickly - you can change your body for the better. But if you have tried and failed before to make the improvements you want because you've become disheartened or struggled with motivation, there is one sure-fire way of keeping your commitment levels higher, and that's doing this plan with a friend. Training with a partner is a proven way to keep you engaged, motivated and positive, so ask someone to join you on your fat-loss journey.

The old saying goes fail to prepare and prepare to fail. And that couldn't be truer with this plan. Luckily, being prepared is easy to do and will make a big difference to your life, lowering stress levels and making your more motivated. All you need to do is make sure you "book in" your three weekly workouts just like another important appointment. You can also prepare your breakfasts and lunches the previous night to make sure you always have a healthy-eating option to keep your body burning fat!

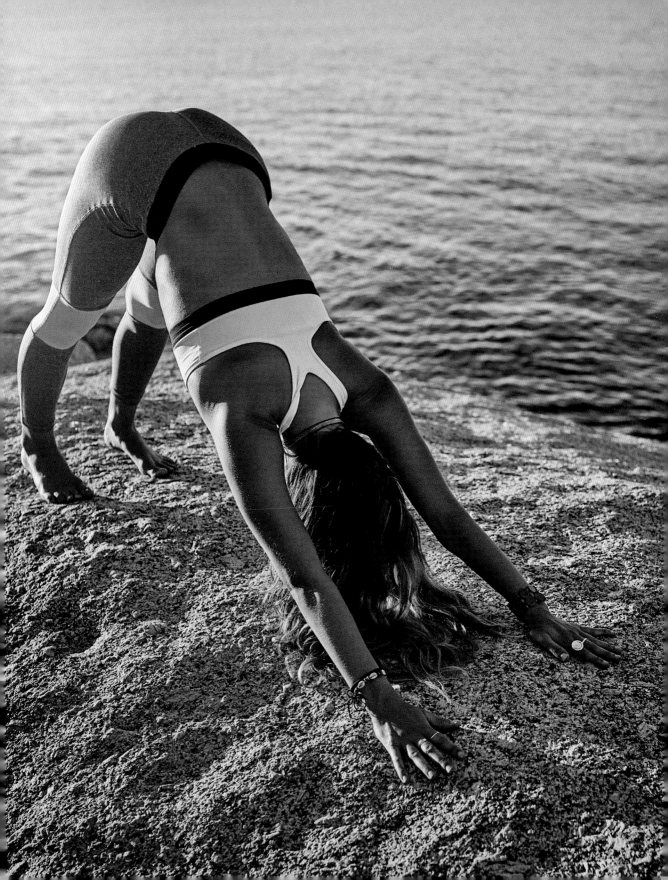

Sleep sounder tonight!

Get high-quality restorative sleep every night to transform how you look and feel

There's supposed to be something very impressive about getting by with very little sleep. We hear highly successful people who get by with only four or five hours a night described as "superhuman". But there is nothing big or clever about surviving on very little sleep. For people who are not natural "short-sleepers" (thought to be just 2% of the population), poor and disturbed sleep is a serious problem. Indeed, a recent UK poll found that only 50% of us are happy with the amount of sleep we get.

Poor sleep has serious consequences for your physical health – it's associated with increased risk of obesity and heart disease – and your mental health. It increases the risk of depression and mood disorders, and impairs decision making, concentration, communication and language skills, among many other problems. But we have the solutions, so read on to learn how to sleep better – starting tonight!

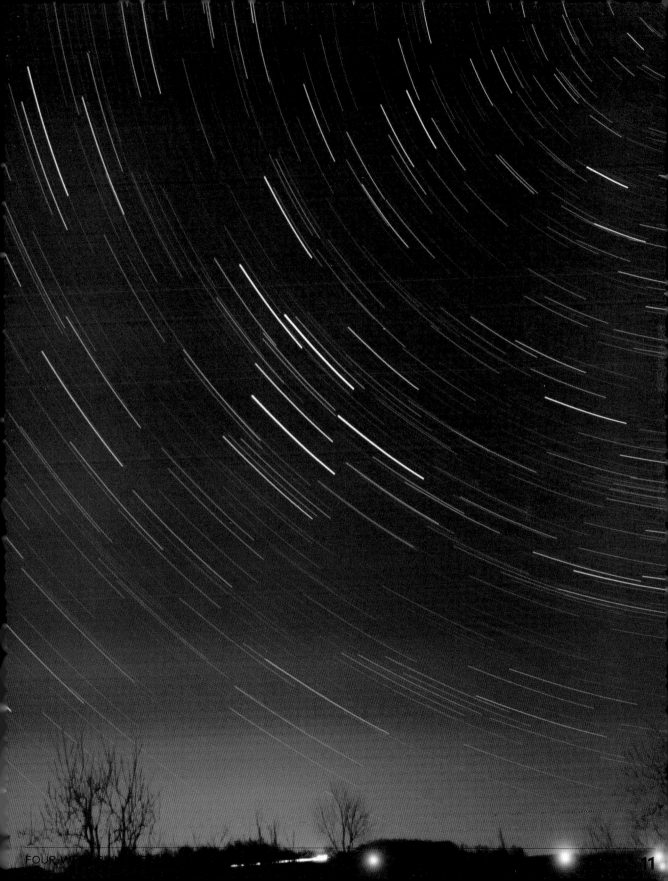

Why is sleep so important? The truth is we still don't have a fully comprehensive answer, but new research is constantly shining the light on some possible explanations. For instance, during the day metabolic "debris" accumulates between the connections in the brain and impairs the ability of nerve cells to communicate. When you sleep the gaps between brain cells open up and spinal fluid flows in, flushing out this junk. If you don't get enough good-quality sleep this process is limited. A recent online experiment that improved sleep among subjects was also successful at reducing depression, anxiety and paranoid thoughts.

7 ways to sleep better

Addressing any sleep issues and improving your sleep quality is one of the most important things you can do for better brain health and better overall health and happiness. Here's how you can sleep better tonight.

❶ Keep cool

A reduction in body temperature is a physiological indicator that it's nearly time for sleep. So if your room or bed is very hot, it makes it far harder to fall asleep and then stay asleep. Have the right tog duvet for the season and use a quiet fan if you need it. Taking a warm bath an hour before bed can also promote the onset of sleep because your body starts cooling down once you step out of the bath.

❷ Get some sun

Exposure to bright, natural light anchors your daily sleep/wake cycle in to a healthy rhythm. Try to get out and spend at least 30 minutes in daylight in the morning or take a half-hour walk after lunch.

❸ Hack your body clock

You may have heard of the circadian rhythm, which is the scientific name for your 24-hour body clock, but what about the ultradian rhythm? This is a 90-minute cycle that repeats throughout the day, and tracking yours can help you identify the best time for you to go to bed.

The ultradian rhythm is remarkably consistent and you can track it by timing your yawns. At the peak of the wave you're at your most alert and it's the perfect time to tackle your to-do list, but 45 minutes later you're at the trough of the wave and most likely to yawn. So, if you yawn around 8:30pm but it's too early to go to bed, you know you're likely to be most sleepy again at 10pm and then 11:30pm. You can then make sure you're in bed by 9:50pm or 11:20pm to get to sleep as quickly as possible.

❹ Put down your phone

Smartphones, tablets and computer screens emit blue light, which is the same wavelength as dawn light, and so is interpreted by your brain as a sign that it's take time wake up, be alert and get active. Try to avoid using your devices for at least an hour before bed or, at the very least, turn on your devices' night-time setting to shift from blue light to red light.

❺ Get blackout curtains

Make sure the room is as dark and quiet as possible and use an eye mask, blackout curtains and ear plugs if you live in or near a noisy environment. Remember that every bit of light or sound pollution can affect your ability to fall asleep and sleep soundly.

❻ Cut back on booze

Although alcohol promotes feelings of tiredness and can help you fall asleep, it disturbs your sleep quality by preventing your brain from entering the deeper, restorative phases of sleep. Try not to drink too much booze before going to bed, and cut back on all drinks: small-hours trips to the loo are very detrimental to a good night's sleep.

❼ Try to relax!

There is no magic number to how much sleep you need. The right amount is enough for you not to feel excessively sleepy during the day. That might be seven hours or nine; we all have different sleep needs. Work out how much you think you need then focus on getting that amount every night.

Quick tip

Good-quality sleep is essential to the health of your brain and body. The link between poor sleep and mood problems, weight gain, diabetes, severe depression and mental illness is clear. Put in the effort to improve your night-time routine and you should improve your physical health, energy, mood and well-being – not just this week or this month, but for years to come!

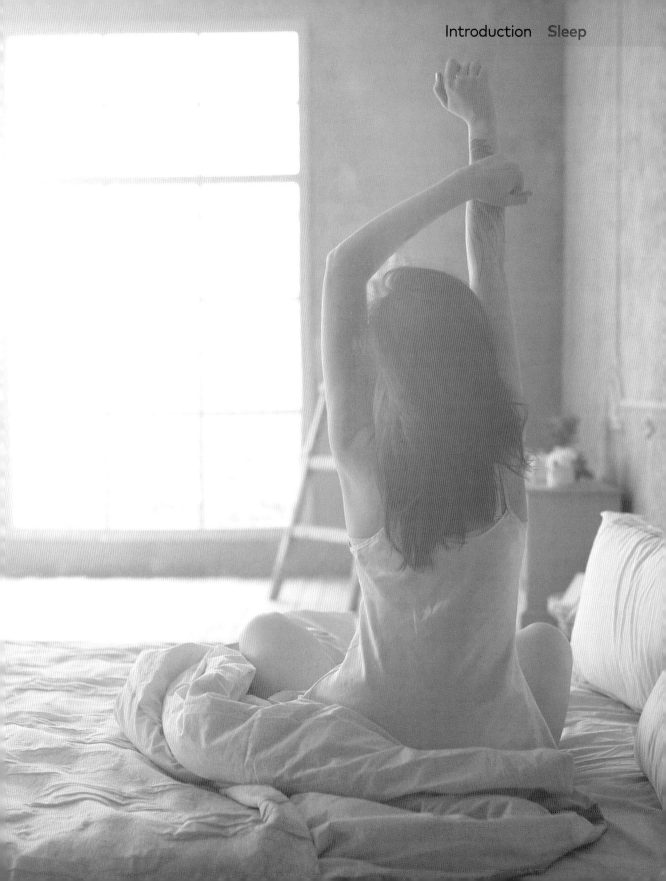

10 steps to building better life habits

Lose weight and live happier with these smart, simple and sustainable lifestyle adjustments

Almost all our behaviours take the form of a habit. Some of these regular routines are great: brushing your teeth is important for avoiding a toothless old age; and making your partner a cup of tea first thing demonstrates appreciation and deepens your bond. But other habits are not so beneficial: hitting the snooze button every morning means you always end up rushing and arrive at work already stressed.

So we all have lots of habits that either enhance or impede our lives, but the good news is there's always the opportunity to break unhelpful habits and create new, beneficial ones.

Establishing good habits reduces the number of decisions you have to make each day, freeing up brainpower for more important tasks. It also reduces the amount of firefighting you have to do fixing problems created by bad habits. Research shows there are some habits that bring a wealth of physical and mental health benefits – and you'll find them over the page!

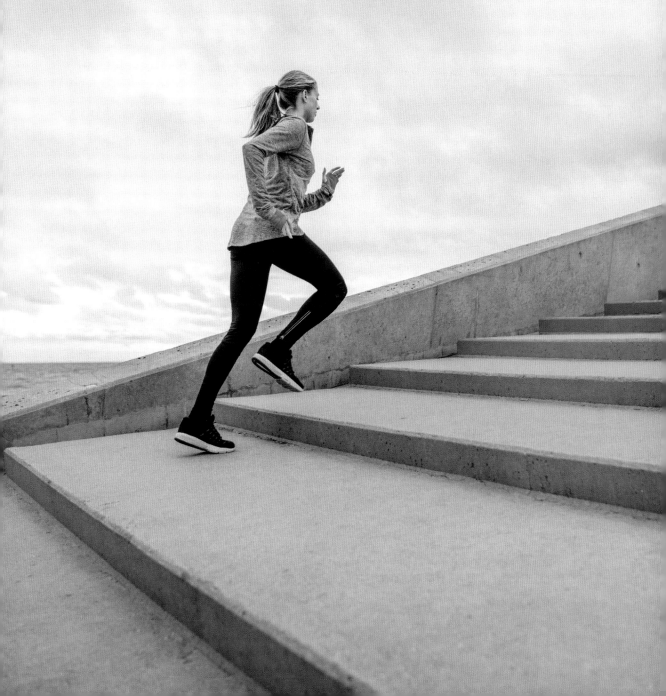

ONE
Be more active

The physical and mental benefits of exercise are so numerous and well established that if exercise were a pill, we'd all be trying to stockpile it. As well as helping you lose body fat and increase lean body mass, exercise also protects the long-term health of the brain in two main ways.

Aerobic activity, such as running, swimming and cycling, increases blood flow to the brain, which brings with it oxygen and nutrients that the brain needs to stay in good working order.

Resistance training, such as bodyweight exercise or lifting dumbbells increases the production of compounds in the brain that protect nerve cells from dying, and promotes the growth of new neural connections. A better-connected brain is faster and more efficient and this extra connectivity, if continued over a long period of time, can protect against the loss of brain volume as we age.

But physical activity isn't only running or doing press-ups: the habit of simply moving more often is linked to longevity and better brain function as we age. If you can start getting into the habit of going for a 20- or 30-minute walk every lunchtime you will make significant strides to improve your health and well-being.

TWO
Eat more veg

From a nutrition perspective eating more greens is probably the single most important new habit you can forge to enhance your health. Veggies are packed with vitamins, minerals, fibre and other compounds such as phytochemicals that have numerous health-boosting qualities. You should be eating a fist-sized portion of veggies with every meal as an absolute minimum.

It's also important to eat a wide range of veggies, because each type and colour contains different combinations of essential nutrients. If you don't like certain vegetables, experiment with different cooking methods or adding different spices or oils to make them more palatable.

THREE
Drink more water

Staying hydrated has repeatedly been shown to improve physical and mental well-being and performance. Research has found people encouraged to drink more water felt less fatigued, had better focus and improved mood, and felt less tired – all factors that promote a sense of well-being. Aim for around two litres a day, but more if you exercise or if it's hot and humid, and carry a water bottle around with you so it's easy to keep drinking all day long.

FOUR
Be more mindful

Getting into the habit of focusing your attention on what's happening in the here and now can lower stress levels, stop you feeling overwhelmed, and improve productivity. A regular mindfulness practice can also reduce inflammation, induce calm and even protect brain health. If you're new to the practice of mindfulness, start with just being more mindful at mealtimes, which means eating in a peaceful and tranquil setting (so not in front of the television or scrolling through your smartphone!) and taking the time to savour and properly chew each mouthful of food. Doing this has been shown to improve the digestion process, so you get more nutrients out of your food, and can help prevent over-eating.

FIVE
Be more grateful

It is so easy to get into the habit of complaining about the things that we don't have or that have gone wrong. It is important to face certain realities, but we need to be careful not to overemphasise the negatives to the detriment of all the good things we have going on.

Simply writing down one thing you're grateful for each day is a genuinely powerful tool for rebalancing your attention and focusing more on the good things in life.

SIX
Connect more

It isn't being dramatic to say loneliness kills. Despite a dizzying array of "social" media platforms many people find they are more isolated and disconnected than ever. Loneliness increases your risk of heart attack, depression and cognitive decline. When people look back on their lives in old age one of the biggest regrets is neglecting relationships, and research shows the people who live longest have cultivated close relationships and are part of stable communities.

Get into the habit of prioritising your relationships. Even if you have to schedule phone calls or make arrangements weeks in advance, it's worth the effort because in-person contact with people who matter to you pays huge dividends to your well-being.

SEVEN
Open up more

There are serious physiological consequences to bottling up your feelings. Not only does it increase dissatisfaction and unhappiness, but holding on to negative emotions can increase inflammation in the body, which is associated with a number of health risks from depression to heart disease. Get into the habit of saying how you feel as soon as you can – you'll be protecting your health, as well as helping prevent the resentment and misunderstandings that harm relationships. If you find it difficult to say how you feel or are in the habit of putting on a brave face, talking to an impartial professional can give you the skills and confidence to be more open.

EIGHT
Be more organised

Are you always running for the train or ignoring bills until they're sent in red ink? Does the word "deadline" conjure up images of caffeine-fuelled all-nighters? If so you need to get more organised, because doing so will reduce your everyday stress levels to make becoming healthier and happier far easier. It's as simple as putting out your work clothes and packing a gym bag the night before, or planning and cooking your meals in advance. It might take a week to get used to these new habits, but once they've taken hold you'll never look back!

 Quick tip Habit change is hard, even when we know it will do us the power of good in the long run, and it takes time and effort to break established routines and rewire your brain to the better way of doing things. Start small, breaking the beneficial habit down into smaller steps and take just one step at a time. And give yourself a break – it's not easy but it will be worth it!

NINE
Get a hobby

For many of us work is something we have to do to enjoy the rest of our lives. Maybe one day you could see whether your personal and professional interests could overlap, but for now it's vital to remember that your job is not your identity, nor is it the extent of your capabilities. Explore that hobby that's always interested you: learn to dance, play an instrument, learn a language, try something you think you'll love. Don't have enough time? Watch an hour less TV a night and now you do! Your new hobby will give you far more satisfaction and ultimately lead to greater happiness.

TEN
Sort your sleep

Skimping on sleep will make you tired, unproductive, depressed, fat and sick – and it'll shorten your life. Developing better bedtime and sleep habits, as you discovered on the previous pages, will make a phenomenal difference to every single part of your life.

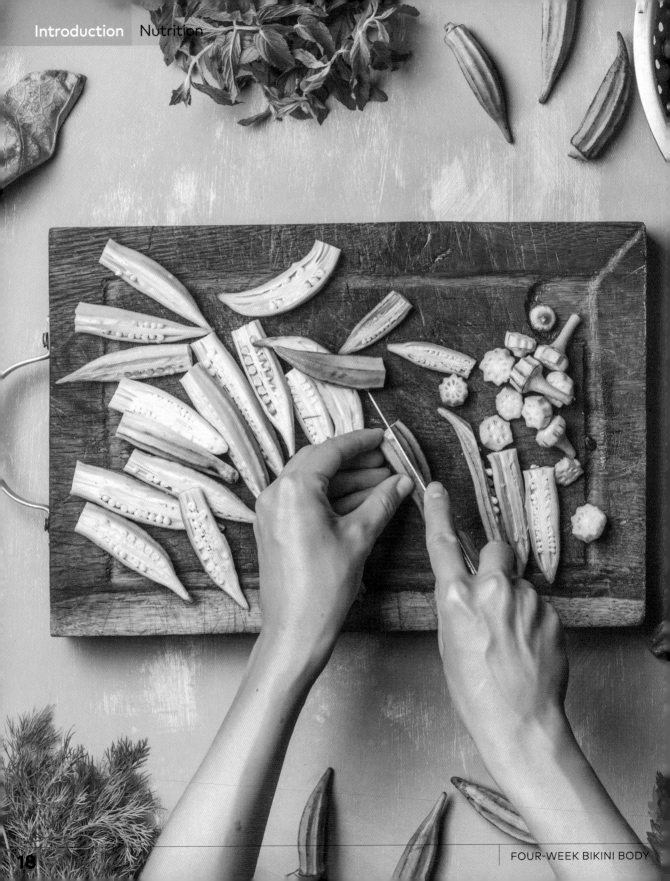

Eat for a lean and strong body

Read on to discover the quick and easy ways to eat well!

In the pursuit of building your best-ever body, what you do in the kitchen is just as important as what you do in the gym, or in whichever space you work out. Why? Because you need to feed your body all the essential nutrients it needs to burn fat while also sculpting leaner and more defined muscles. Read on to discover the smart and sustainable approaches you can follow to eat for a better body!

Fuel your better body mission!

Start eating smarter to burn off stubborn body fat and sculpt a stronger and leaner body to look and feel better than ever

You are what you eat, and when your goal is to strip away fat whilst toning and defining your muscles to build your best-ever body, what you eat really matters. That doesn't mean that you must dramatically cut back on calories, give up certain foods or entire food groups, or even go on some crazy juice diet. Indeed, the only way to lose weight and - crucially - keep it off for good is to follow a smart and sustainable approach to eating.

Don't worry if that sounds too simplistic to work, or if you don't know where to start: in this chapter you'll discover why low-calorie diets make you fatter and sadder; what's in the food you eat and why it's vital to eat a varied and balanced diet; how to be more present at mealtimes (and why doing so will help you shift fat faster); the simple mind-tricks to help you stop overeating for good, and more so you can start eating for a leaner and healthier body, starting right now!

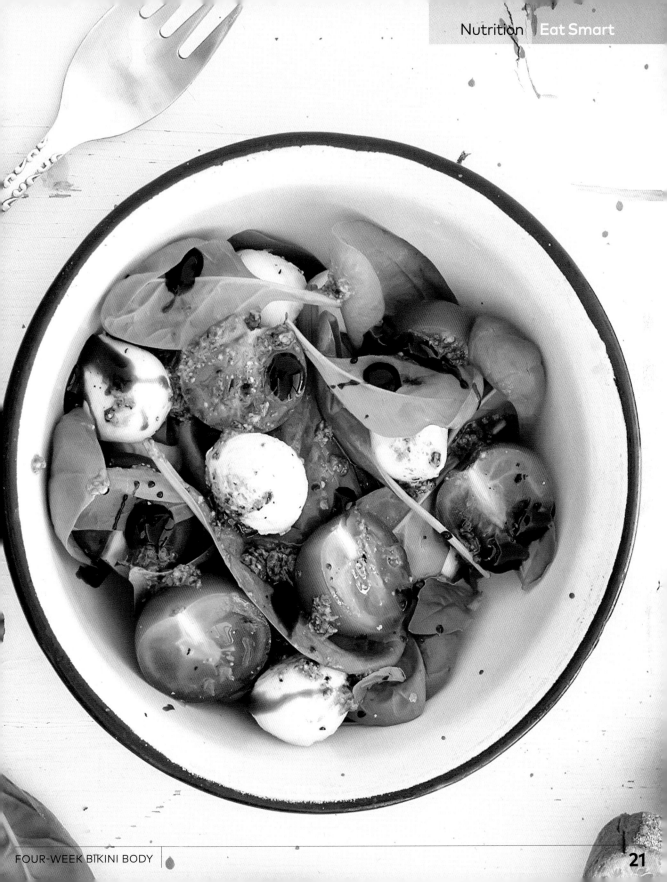

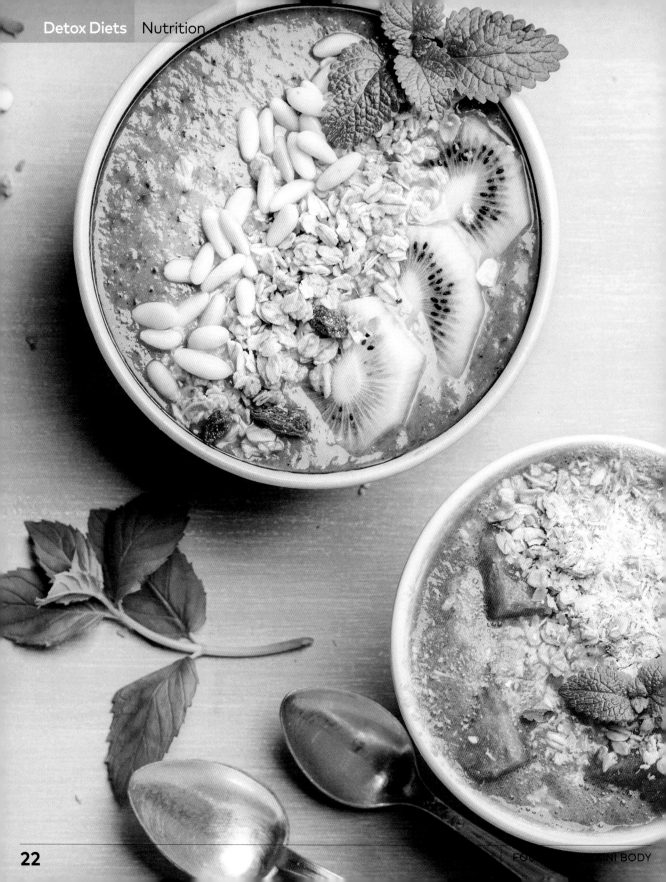

Ditch the detox diet!

Want to lose fat fast? Here's why "quick-fix" diets are the worst thing you can do!

We've been all there: waking up the morning after the night before. Or the morning after the weekend before! Perhaps you drank too much, ate too much, or had too much of something that disagrees with you. For many people, it's at this moment – or when they face the mirror, or get on the bathroom scale, or struggle to buckle their belt – that they start thinking about a diet.

Most people want quick results: you feel bad now and want to feel better asap. But while quick-fix diets – whether they're called a "detox", a "cleanse", a "metabolic reset" or any other attention-grabbing name – promise instant results, they never work for long. Even worse, they'll make you fatter and unhappier in the long run.

How do I lose – or gain – weight?
Before we get to why quick-fix diets are so dangerous it's important to understand how we gain and lose weight. In theory, weight loss is simple. It's based on the Energy Balance Equation, which says that to lose weight you must consume less energy – in other words, fewer calories from food – than you burn.

We expend energy through simply being alive (our bodies burn calories at rest to keep us alive, at what's known as the basal metabolic rate or BMR), and also through everyday activities, exercise and excretion. Over time if we eat fewer calories than we burn, we lose weight; if we eat more calories than we burn, we gain weight.

This concept is important to understand because it's how all diets work. It doesn't matter if you're only eating "superfoods", having one meal a day or ten, or eat standing on your head (don't do that) – you'll lose weight only if you consume less energy than you expend. But that doesn't mean all diets are equal in helping you lose weight, or improving your health and happiness! Keep reading to discover why "detox diets" are so bad for both your body and your brain.

5 reasons detox diets are so dangerous

Here's why quick-fix diets damage your health and make you fatter!

PROBLEM 1

You mess up your fluid balance

Why is this bad? Many quick-fix or fad diets "work" because when you first start restricting your food intake or cut out certain nutrients to reduce your daily calorie consumption, you will lose weight. A big problem is that it's not fat that you've lost – it's water. And that's the last thing you want to happen.

This is one reason detox diets are so incredibly dangerous. They can negatively affect your body's fluid and salt (better known as electrolyte) balance, which means you can lose a lot of water and salts very quickly. Disrupting fluid and electrolyte balance will result in dehydration, which will make you look, feel and perform far worse than normal.

Take things too far and these dangers become much more serious because your body depends on fluid and electrolyte balance for maintaining the rhythm of your heart, as well as many other very important functions.

So if you're ever tempted to try one of those so-called "detox diets", remember that you might see a lower number on the bathroom scale after a few days but any weight lost is probably water, rather than that body fat you really want to shift. And remember it's likely to make you feel tired, dehydrated and miserable – and that's about as far from living a healthier and happier life as you can be.

PROBLEM 2

You starve your body of nutrients

Why is this bad? Almost all quick-fix diets are based on severely restricting your daily calorie intake by cutting out specific types of foods or eliminating food groups entirely.

This means that these diets don't provide some, or even many, of the essential nutrients your body needs to function at its best – whether that's fats, protein or vitamins and minerals. So they will dramatically affect how "healthy" you look and feel.

You may suffer physical signs, such as dry, pale or dull skin, aching joints and muscles, feelings of lethargy and weakness, or trouble falling and staying asleep, as well as a wide range of mental symptoms, not limited to constant hunger, low energy and constant fatigue, bad moods, and dire levels of focus, motivation and concentration.

All you will think about is food and your next meal, not to mention that pit-of-your-stomach disappointment about what that next meal is going to be!

This will make you feel absolutely awful in the short term and cause you to question whether all these negative side effects are worth it. (They're not.) But it has an even more serious impact on your long-term health, fitness and general well-being.

PROBLEM 3
Your metabolism slows down

Why is this bad? Your body's job, evolutionarily speaking, is to stop you starving to death – a very real risk until relatively recently. So your body pays very close attention to how much you're eating.

When you suddenly start eating less your body makes adjustments to prevent starvation. Your metabolism slows down to conserve energy, and many other changes occur. Your digestive tract moves food through more slowly to extract as much energy and as many nutrients as possible (which can cause digestive issues, such as bloating or constipation); your repair and recovery processes slow down so you don't heal as fast; and there's a reduced production of important hormones, including the primary sex hormones oestrogen, progesterone and testosterone.

When your metabolism slows, your body decides you need even less energy to survive, which means you now must further reduce your calorie intake from food to get into that calorie deficit to lose weight! This creates a vicious cycle in which your body, over time, requires fewer and fewer calories to function, making it harder to lose weight even when you're eating far less than before. This is really bad for your weight loss ambition. Why? Keep reading.

PROBLEM 4
Your appetite roars back

Why is this bad? Have you ever wondered what makes you feel hungry? Or full? Appetite is controlled by a series of feedback loops in the digestive system and the brain. There are also sensors in our fat cells that tell our brain how full our fat stores are. If there's a lack of food being eaten, these feedback loops and sensors compensate by making you really hungry. The "if you're standing between me and the fridge I can't be held responsible for my actions" kind of hungry!

No matter how strong your willpower and motivation, your brain's "don't starve" system is always stronger.

Eventually you quit the diet (because it's unsustainable and you're miserable) and resume eating normally. But you now need fewer calories than before because of your slower metabolism, so you gain back the weight you lost – and more – because your brain is sending all the excess energy to fill up your fat stores in an effort to make sure you don't "starve" again. You'll think about food more often – and hence eat more too. This is a major reason so many people end up yo-yo dieting and gain body fat rather than losing it.

PROBLEM 5
You get stuck in a vicious cycle

Why is this bad? There are many physiological problems caused by quick-fix diets, but one of the biggest is the damaging habits that they cause people to adopt.

To lose weight and keep it off, you must make some simple and sustainable habit changes. We'll get to how you can do that really easily soon, but first here are some of the worst habits that are forged by quick-fix diets.

- You learn to either be "on" a diet or "off" it – there is nothing in between
- You only ever experience a very short period of weight loss "success", if any
- You experience long periods of "failure", and feelings of guilt or frustration that add to your unhappiness
- You start to develop a damaging relationship with food and think obsessively about eating
- You forget how to "trust" your body to know how it's really feeling, and don't trust yourself to make smart food choices
- You end up in one of two equally bad scenarios: either living a life adhering to a very strict set of eating rules, or suffering from a complete loss of control over your diet and your life

What's in your food?

Here's a guide to the major and minor components in the food you eat – and why they're so important

Every single thing we eat is a combination of different compounds. Most natural, unprocessed food consists primarily of water: a banana is 75% water, a potato is 79% water and a chicken breast, which most people think of as pure protein, can be up to 75% water. But this isn't actually that surprising when you consider you are around 70% water – so you're more H_2O than anything else!

After water the next most common compound in natural foods will be a macronutrient – there are three of them – or a combination of macronutrients along with certain micronutrients. Turn the page to find out more.

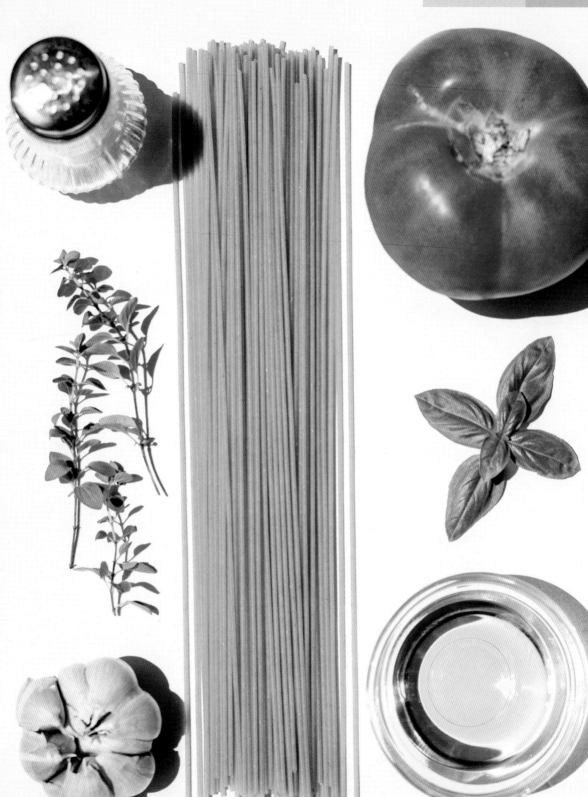

What are macronutrients?
Macronutrients are the three main groups of chemical compounds that make up the food we eat. They are protein, fats and carbohydrates.

What are micronutrients?
Micronutrients are chemical compounds such as vitamins, minerals and phytonutrients (plant-based nutrients) in food. They are found in much smaller quantities than macronutrients, and we only need them in very small amounts.

MACRONUTRIENTS
Protein
After water, most of what makes you, well, *you* is made from proteins, and all proteins are made from amino acids. There are many types of amino acid, most of which your body can manufacture itself when required, but there are nine amino acids your body can't synthesise. They're called "essential amino acids" and you must get them from food. Most foods contain at least small (or "trace") amounts of protein, but these are some of the most protein-rich foods.

Animal sources
- poultry (chicken, turkey, duck, goose) and eggs
- red meat (beef, pork, lamb)
- wild game (venison, rabbit, pheasant)
- fish and shellfish
- dairy (milk, cheese, yogurt)

Plant sources
- beans and legumes
- tofu, tempeh and other soy products
- nuts and seeds (though these are generally much higher in fat than protein)
- some grains such as quinoa, amaranth and wild rice (though these are much higher in carbohydrates than protein)

How much do I need?
A good target is about 0.8g-1g of protein per kilogram of bodyweight per day, but you may need more if you're active, older, pregnant or breastfeeding, or ill or injured.

Carbohydrates
There are many types of carbohydrates and they're mainly found in plant-based foods. Some carbs are very simple molecules, such as sugars, which are the most basic form. Others are much more complicated and are called complex carbohydrates. Starches, which are found in potatoes and beans, are one type of complex carb, as is fibre.

The more "simple" the carbohydrate the easier it is to digest and absorb. In general, when eating for better health and fitness you want to prioritise consuming complex carbohydrates because they are slower-digesting and more nutrient-rich than simple carbs.

Our bodies can't completely break down some types of complex carbs, such as insoluble fibre or resistant starch, but the bacteria in our gut love it and make other beneficial compounds from it. Fibre and resistant starch are often known as "prebiotics": they're food sources that nourish our "good" gut bacteria. Fibre also helps move things through our intestinal tract.

Higher-fibre foods include fruits and vegetables, whole grains, beans and legumes, and nuts and seeds, and resistant starch is found in beans, green bananas, and many other plant-based foods.

Water
Make sure you're drinking enough to stay fit and focused

We are about 70% water and can't live long without it. Regulating thirst and maintaining the balance of fluids and electrolytes are two of your body's most vital tasks. We take in water through drinking, obviously, but also through eating fluid-rich fruits and veg, and we lose it through breathing, sweating and excretion.

You've probably heard you need to drink eight glasses of water per day, but there's no evidence to support that. There's also no reason to be peeing "clear" urine: a light yellow colour is fine.

There are simple ways to avoid dehydration: drink a big glass of water as soon as you wake up; pay more attention to thirst; drink more during exercise or in hot or humid conditions; choose water as your go-to drink (instead of alcohol or caffeinated drinks); and check your urine colour (the darker it is, the more dehydrated you are). If you often forget to drink enough water – you may notice you feel mentally and physically tired – fill up a water bottle at the beginning of the day, keep it close and take a big gulp every time you look at it!

Best sources of fibre and micronutrient-rich carbs

- Sweet and starchy vegetables (winter squashes, beetroot)
- Starchy tubers (potatoes, sweet potatoes, yams)
- Whole grains (rice, wheat, oats)
- Beans and legumes
- Fruit

How much do I need?

That depends on myriad factors, including your activity levels: you need more carbs if you are physically active and/or trying to build muscle. While some people do benefit from a lower-carb diet, most people look, feel and perform better from eating at least some carbs, especially the nutrient-rich, higher-fibre types.

> If you eat processed foods you will consume substances that are technically edible, such as preservatives, binders and colouring agents, but these are not really "food".

Fats

The main three types of dietary fat are saturated, monounsaturated and polyunsaturated (see below). They differ from one another by the number and frequency of the carbon atoms that bond them, but we don't need to worry about that! You just need to know that fats are an essential macronutrient and you need to consume them for optimal health (it's yet another reason why very low-fat "detox diets" make you look and feel so bad!).

How much do I need?

Most people do best with 25-35% of their total daily calories coming from a wide variety of healthy fat sources. Omega-3 fatty acids, particularly EPA and DHA, are special types of fats found in oily fish, seafood and some plant sources. They can help you lose weight, boost brain function, reduce inflammation, and improve both your physical and mental health – they're all-round performers!

You may have noticed that processed cooking oils, margarine and cooking sprays don't appear here and with good reason! Most "long life" cooking oils and margarines are heavily processed and contain types of fat called "trans fats" that aren't found in nature, so your body doesn't know how to process them. Research increasingly suggests trans fats contribute to many health problems.

MICRONUTRIENTS

Vitamins and minerals come in many forms and what we think of as a "vitamin" or a "mineral" is actually a group of molecules that are chemically similar, but sufficiently different to do different jobs in the body. For example "vitamin A" is actually a family of molecules, and the carotenoid forms of vitamin A (such as beta-carotene) are water-soluble, found mainly in plants (such as carrots), and not very well absorbed; while the retinoid forms of vitamin A are fat-soluble, found mostly in animal foods (such as egg yolks) and are well absorbed.

We absorb minerals such as calcium, iron and magnesium from dairy and meat better than from leafy greens, which come in harder-to-digest forms. This is one reason why it's important to eat a wide variety of foods: each food has a unique chemical "fingerprint" of micronutrients that contributes to our good health.

You may think taking a multi-vitamin or multi-mineral supplement helps you avoid deficiencies, but taking more vitamin and/or mineral pills is not usually better or healthier. Instead, focus on improving the quality and variety of your food choices so that you get your vitamins and minerals in the form that nature intended.

The 3 types of fat

Most fat sources contain more than one type of dietary fat, but these foods are particularly high in one type

Saturated fats	Monounsaturated fats	Polyunsaturated fats
• Butter and high-fat dairy (eg cheese)	• Avocado	• Many types of seeds such as flax, chia, sesame and sunflower seeds
• Most animal fats	• Olives and olive oil	
• Coconut and coconut oil	• Peanuts	• Oily fish such as salmon, herring, and mackerel
• Egg yolk	• Many types of nuts, such as pecans and almonds	
• Cacao butter		

How to stop overeating!

It can be easy to eat too much despite not wanting to, which makes losing fat harder. Here's why it happens, and how you can stop it

Whether it's a birthday, a holiday, socialising with friends or just a Friday night with a takeaway pizza, all of us at some point eat too much. But for some of us this happens more often than we'd like. Here we'll look at some of the main reasons that can trigger over-eating, and then we'll provide some really simple strategies you can use to overcome them.

FACTOR 1

Your prehistoric brain

The first thing to understand about overeating is that most of it isn't your fault – at least, not consciously. Evolution has ensured that our brains pay a lot of attention to food; that our brains prefer sweet, fatty and savoury foods that are high in energy; and that we tend to eat more rather than less, in case a famine is around the corner.

This was a life-saving strategy until very recently in human history. But we now live in a world where food, especially processed food high in calories but low in nutrients, is tasty, cheap and accessible, and hard to quit eating once you start. Food manufacturers know what our hungry brains like and purposely make processed foods that appeal to them.

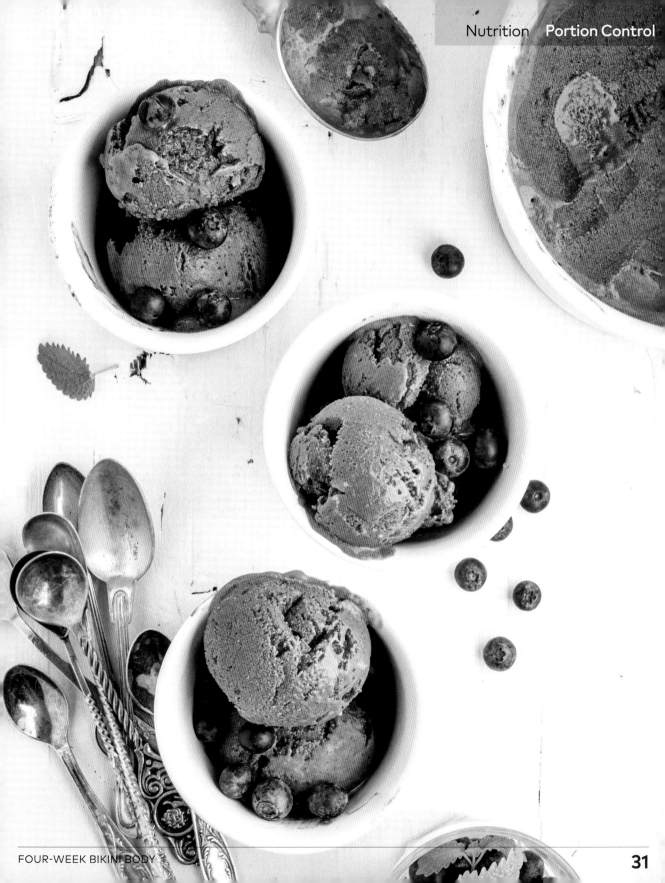

FACTOR 2
Your food triggers

We make hundreds of food decisions a day, but we aren't aware of most of them. We rarely consciously choose what and how to eat. Instead, we tend to go on autopilot and rely on routines, habits and what's easiest.

We eat in our cars, on the train, walking to work, at our desks and on the go, usually without stopping and thinking about it. When we see or smell food we just grab it and eat it, and we rarely slow down, sit down and experience it mindfully with full awareness. We're often mentally or physically tired, which makes it even harder to make smart food choices, which is why achieving mealtime mindfulness is so important.

And as a woman your natural hormonal fluctuations may affect your hunger, appetite and ability to control your eating.

FACTOR 3
Your stress levels

Stress and emotional well-being are the two other big factors behind overeating.

Most of us feel some level of stress in our lives, as well as difficult emotions such as loneliness, anxiety, guilt and fatigue. We may feel over-stimulated from stress or under-stimulated from boredom. Food is a very effective "medication" for stress, difficult emotions and over- or under-stimulation. At least, it is temporarily.

Then, of course, we might feel more stressed or worse after we've overeaten. And so the cycle begins again.

FACTOR 4
Your self-imposed food rules

Many people try to "fix" overeating with a strict diet or eating rules such as "No food after 7pm" or "No sugar ever again".

Unfortunately, as you now know, these restrictions backfire. You soon resent following such rules, or feel deprived. If you've reduced what you eat dramatically, your body responds by turning up the appetite signals and attention to food cues, so food becomes really, really appealing.

Eventually, people go right back to overeating and then they feel even worse. The cycle repeats, over and over, and each time it becomes harder and harder to break.

FACTOR 5
Your regular routine

We all have routines and for many of us, there are certain times when we are more likely to overeat. These are the most common…

- Weekends
- Evenings
- After work
- Parties and other social events
- After the kids have – finally – gone to bed
- Watching TV

How to stop overeating

Looking back over the list of factors above, two things jump out as the biggest causes of overeating on a day-to-day basis: eating quickly and eating while distracted. So there are two really simple first steps you could take to deal with these:

- Slow down the speed at which you eat.
- Pay attention to the foods you are eating.

Here are some other contributing factors and some strategies you could use to overcome them.

Contributing factor #1
You see "food cues" everywhere

Potential strategies
- Look at your environment and routines to see where you can adjust, control and/or eliminate those cues.
- Make it easier to eat healthy foods and harder to get hold of unhealthy ones. So if you have a "trigger" food, don't keep it in your house.

Contributing factor #2
You fall into automatic behaviours without realising

Potential strategies
- Slow down. Pause before you make choices. Ask yourself, "Is this the smartest choice I can make right now? What might be better?"
- Sit at a table to eat and focus as much as possible on the actual act of eating.

Contributing factor #3
You always eat too quickly

Potential strategies
- Eat slowly and chew your food for longer.
- Put down your cutlery between mouthfuls.
- Take a breath between each bite.
- Try to really taste and savour the food.

Contributing factor #4
You turn to food when stressed or emotional

Potential strategies
- Take a few deep breaths before you make a food choice or start eating.
- Ask yourself, "Am I feeling hungry right now?" Pause and identify whether you might be thinking or experiencing another feeling.
- Seek help with managing stress and emotions from a therapist or counsellor.

Contributing factor #5
You impose strict eating rules on yourself

Potential strategies
- Recognise that restrictive rules, or following a strict diet, is not a solution to overeating – indeed it may even increase and worsen your overeating habit in the long run.

Other strategies
As we discussed earlier in this chapter, it's not helpful to label individual foods with rigid moral labels such as "good versus bad" or "clean versus cheating". Instead use categories such as...

- "eat more often" or "eat less often"
- "works well for me" or "doesn't work well for me"
- "makes me feel better" or "makes me feel worse"

Instead of using external rules, work on learning your own internal signals of hunger and fullness, and don't feel failure, frustration or shame after an overeating episode: treat yourself with compassion. Look at each overeating episode as an opportunity to learn more about your triggers so that you can keep finding better ways to overcome them next time.

Start to ask yourself more questions about your daily and weekly routines and identify your triggers, then write down some solutions to overcome them. For instance, where and when are you less likely to overeat? What works well about those situations? Can you do or get more of that? Conversely, where and when are you more likely to overeat? How can you disrupt those situations or do something differently?

Keep moving forwards!
As you learn to change your habits you'll make mistakes. That's normal! Changing behaviours takes time so if you do overeat don't beat yourself up: this will only make it worse. Try to use these responses instead.

- Stay positive! Focus on what you're doing well and the positive choices you've been making. Most of the time, we're doing better than we realise!
- Recognise it's normal. Many people struggle with overeating. You're not bad or broken!
- Keep learning, and notice what situations and factors make it easier for you to make wiser food choices.
- Think like a scientist! Take notes about what caused you to overeat and what occurred when you did. Analyse that info and look for patterns to identify strategies for the future.
- Reboot asap! Wipe the slate clean and start again, immediately. Every time will get a little bit easier.

Quick tip

The biggest factors behind overeating are speed, distraction and stress. So slow down, breathe and pay attention! Choose natural whole foods such as fruits and vegetables, which make you feel healthy, satisfied and energetic, and try to eat until sated, not stuffed! Take the time to listen to your body's natural hunger and fullness signals, and appreciate the simple act of sitting down and savouring every mouthful.

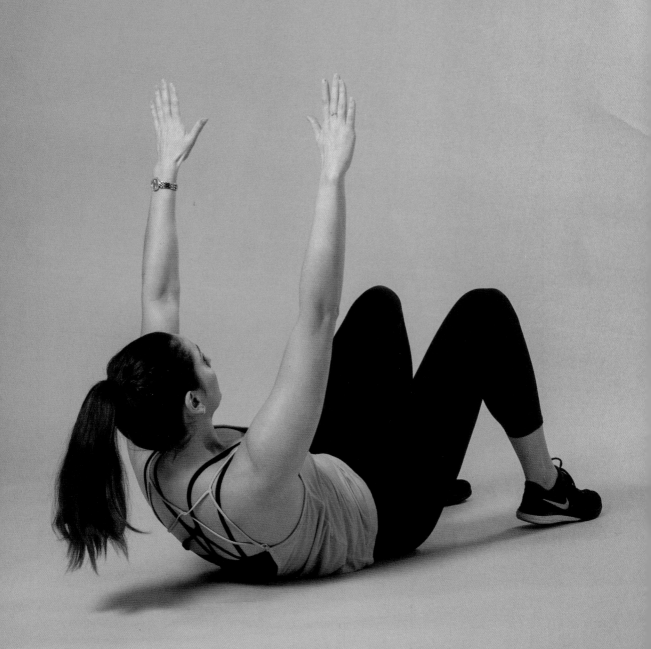

Four weeks to a leaner, stronger you!

You're almost ready to start your own Four-Week Bikini Body journey - but first you need to read the following pages to fully understand how the plan works so you can follow it perfectly. After all, the more you can apply yourself during your workouts, the faster you'll burn fat, the quicker you'll sculpt defined muscles and the greater your four-week results will be!

Workout FAQ

Q
HOW DOES THIS PLAN WORK?

A
This plan is so easy to follow! There are three workouts a week for the next month. Each workout is an eight-move total-body circuit, so you'll do the moves in order, for a certain amount of time and rest between them. This approach is one of the best ways to burn fat and sculpt your muscles. The exercises change after the first fortnight to keep your progress moving in the right direction. All you need to complete each workout is 25 minutes, a little bit of a space, and a big desire to change your body!

Q
WILL THIS PLAN WORK FOR ME?

A
Absolutely! The plan has been designed to keep you progressing every session and every week, so that you're always taking steps in the right direction. Each week the workouts become slightly harder and more challenging, because that's the only way to keep your body from settling into its comfort zone, where it's tough to make big changes to your body. For the best chance of success, make a real effort to stick to the training plan and prioritise getting quality sleep every night to give your body the rest and recovery it needs.

Q
MUST I FOLLOW IT EXACTLY?

A
Consistent effort is crucial to any successful attempt to change your body for the better, so you need to find the time to exercise three times a week for the next four weeks. The circuits in the plan take less than half an hour to complete, so it's not a huge time commitment. Remember, the more closely you can stick to this guide, the more impressive your results will be – and the bigger the change to the way you look and feel will be.

Q
I'VE HAD INJURIES. CAN I STILL DO IT?

A
You should always seek approval from your doctor or medical professional before beginning any new exercise or diet regime, especially if you have had injuries in the past or are currently suffering from injuries or illness. If you have any underlying health concerns at all, check with a qualified expert before you start this plan.

Q
WHAT IF I MISS A SESSION?

A
It's almost inevitable that, at some point over the next month, something will get in the way of your planned training session or stop you from eating the right meal at the right time. It's not the end of the world if you miss a workout so don't give yourself a hard time – but it's vital to get back on track as soon as possible if you want to get into amazing shape. Don't let one missed session turn into two. A consistent approach is the only one that works.

Q
WHAT DO I DO ONCE I'VE DONE IT?

A
The beauty of this plan – in addition to giving you all the tools you need to build a leaner and fitter body – is that once you've completed it (and got into great shape!) you can then start the advanced four-week plan, which starts on p96. While similar in structure to the first plan - it's eight moves per session and three sessions per week – the addition of dumbbells makes these workouts harder and tests your heart, lungs and muscles in new and challenging ways so that your body keeps getting leaner, stronger and healthier!

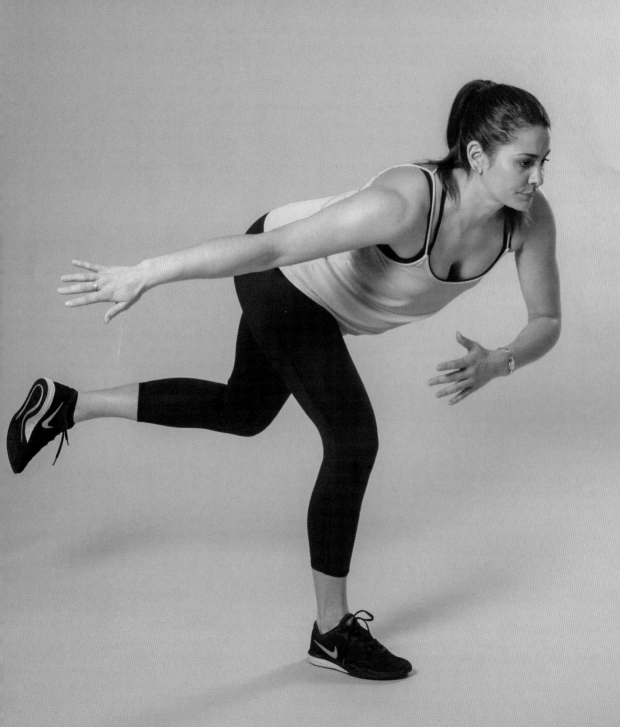

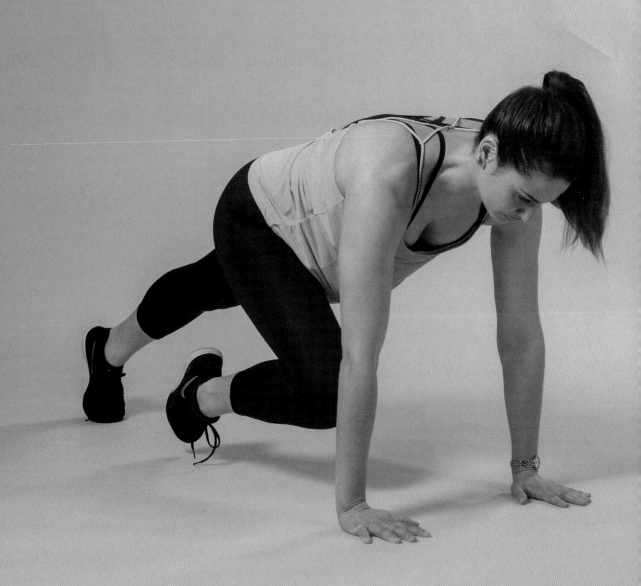

Let's do this!

You're now ready to begin your Four-Week Bikini Body plan. On the next page you'll discover all you need to know and it really couldn't be simpler: each week you'll do three circuit-style sessions. Each workout contains eight moves, which you'll do for a set amount of time, before resting for a set time, and then move on to the next exercise. You get a longer rest at the end of each round, and then you go again!

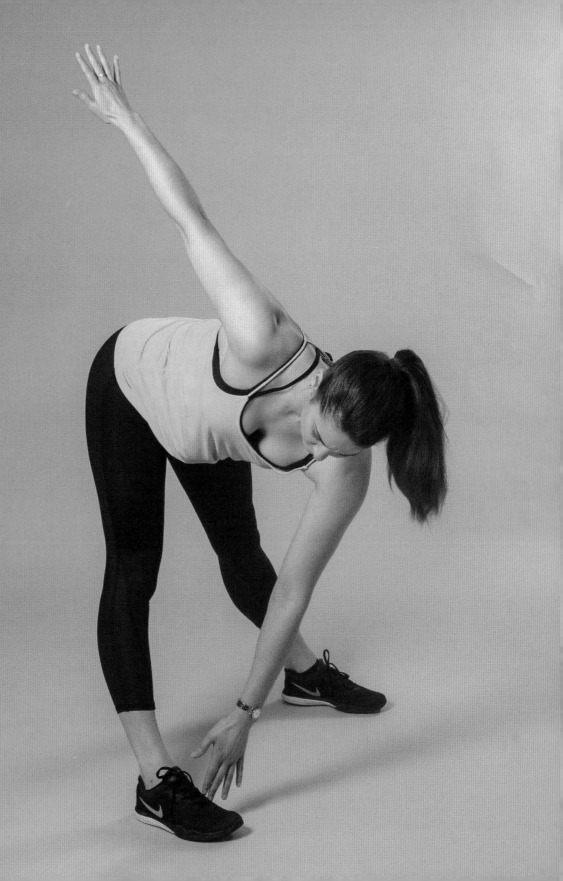

Week 1

Leave a day between each session in this, and every, week

In this first week there's three eight-move total-body circuit sessions. This high-intensity approach will kick-start the fat-burning process and will also sculpt lean and defined muscles - which is exactly what we want! Do the eight moves in order, moving then resting for the durations stated by each move's name - and not a second more or less! Complete the circuit a total of four times and remember to stay hydrated!

1 Squat

TIME 30sec **REST** 30sec

DO 4
CIRCUITS
IN TOTAL

Stand tall with your chest up, abs engaged and arms straight by your sides. Bend your knees to squat down as low as you can, either keeping your hands by your sides or raising them up to shoulder height. Push through your heels to straighten your legs and return to the start position.

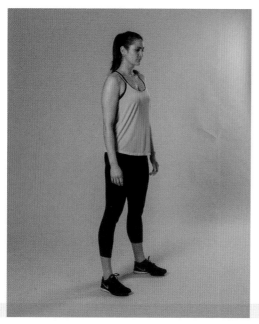
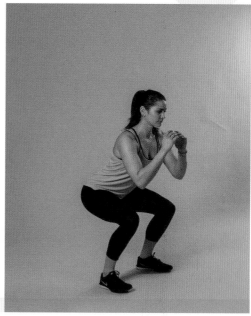

2 Chair dip - bent knees

TIME 30sec **REST** 30sec

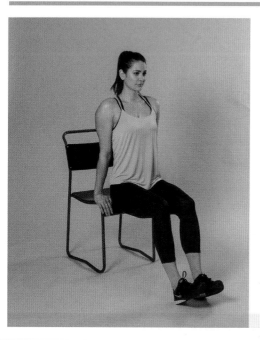
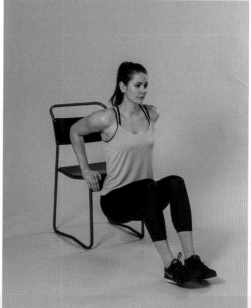

Place your hands on the edge of a chair behind you with your arms straight and knees bent. Keeping your chest up, bend your elbows to lower your bum towards the floor. Go as low as you can, then press back up to straighten your arms and return to the start position.

3 **Side lunge**

Stand tall with your chest up, abs engaged and arms by your sides. Take a big step to your left, then bend your left leg to lunge down. Push through your left foot to return to the start, then repeat by taking a big step to your right. Alternate sides with each rep.

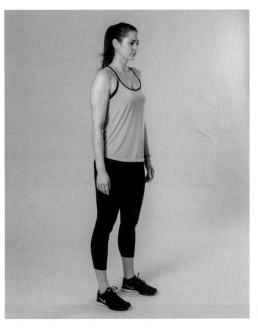
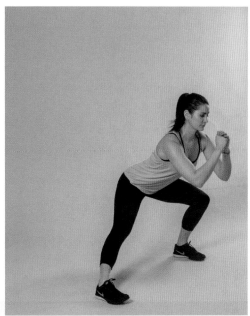

4 **Alternating toe touch**

TIME 30sec **REST** 30sec

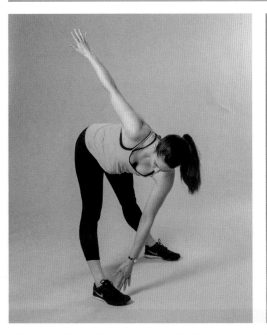
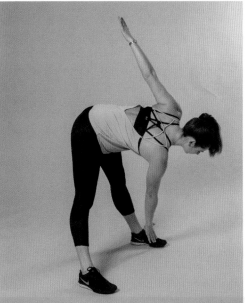

Stand tall with your chest up. Bend down from your hips, trying to keep your legs straight, and touch your right foot with your left hand. Stand back up and repeat, touching your left foot with your right hand. Alternate sides with each rep.

5 Standing sprint

TIME 30sec **REST** 30sec

Stand tall with your chest up and abs engaged. Sprint on the spot, raising your knees as high as possible and swinging your arms back and forth.

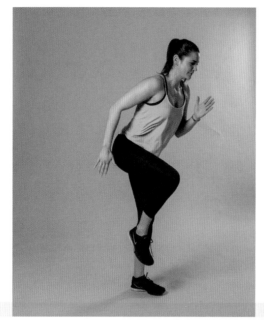
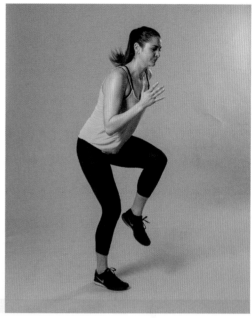

6 Pogo

TIME 30sec **REST** 30sec

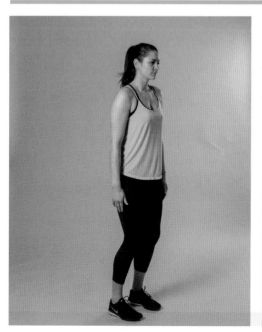
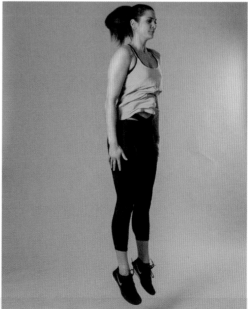

Stand tall with your chest up, abs engaged and arms by your sides. Spring straight up into the air, keeping your arms by your sides. Land on both feet and go straight into the next jump.

7 Bicycles

TIME 30sec **REST** 30sec

Lie on your back with your fingers by your temples and legs straight. Raise your torso, engage your abs, and lift your feet. Crunch up and rotate to one side, bringing your opposite knee in to touch your elbow. Reverse the move to return to the starting position and repeat alternating sides.

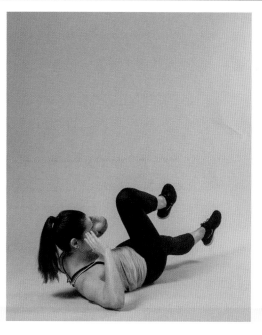
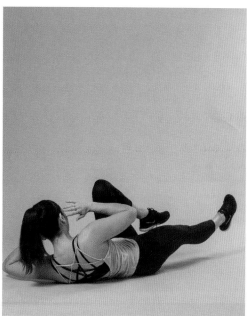

8 Tall plank

TIME 30sec **REST** 2min

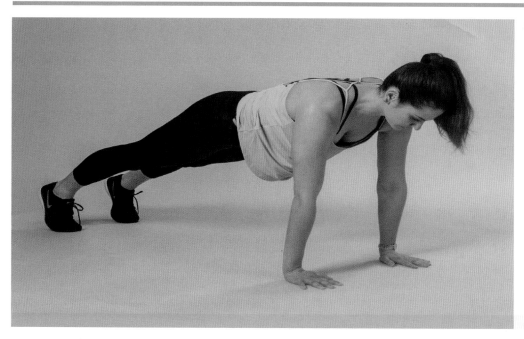

Get into position with your palms on the floor, your wrists underneath your shoulders and your body in a straight line from head to heels. Keep your abs and glutes (bum muscles) engaged to hold this position without letting your hips sag. Keep your breathing controlled and relaxed.

1 Prisoner squat

TIME 40sec **REST** 20sec

DO 4 CIRCUITS IN TOTAL

Stand tall with your chest up, abs engaged and elbows bent with your fingers by your temples. Bend your knees to squat down as low as you can. Push through your heels to straighten your legs and return to the start position.

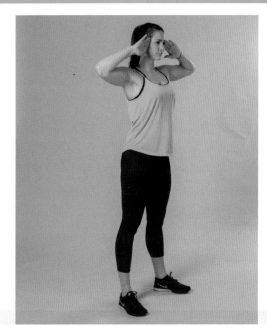
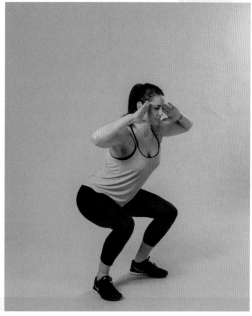

2 Knee press-up

TIME 40sec **REST** 20sec

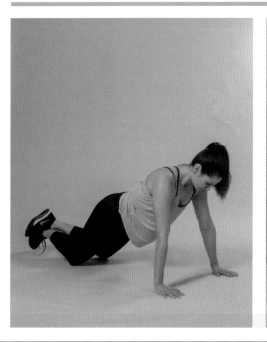
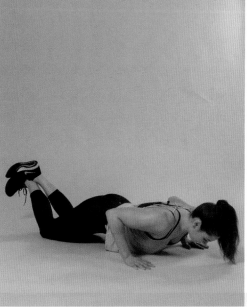

Get on your hands and knees with your bodyweight shifted forwards. Engage your abs and bend your elbows to lower your chest towards the floor. Go as low as you can, then press back up to straighten your arms and return to the start position.

3 Curtsy lunge

TIME 40sec **REST** 20sec

Stand tall with your chest up, your abs engaged and your hands by your sides. Keeping your chest up place one foot behind the other, then bend both knees to lunge down until your back knee almost touches the floor. Push off your rear foot to return to the start position, then repeat, leading with your other leg.

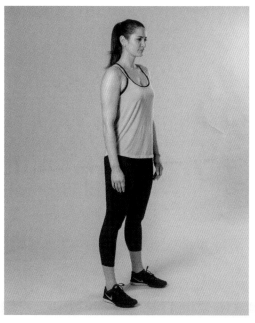
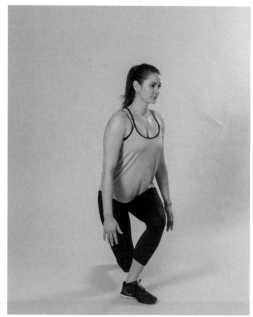

4 RDL

TIME 40sec **REST** 20sec

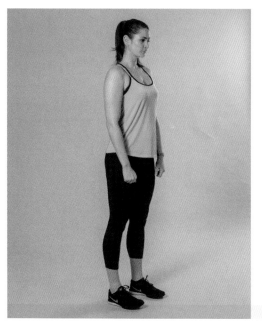
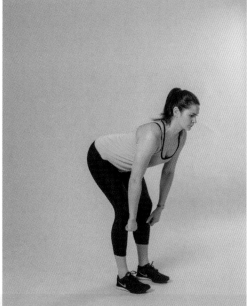

Stand tall with your chest up and abs engaged. With a slight bend in your knees, bend forwards from the hips and reach down the front of your legs, touching your fingertips to them as low down as possible. Stand up to return to the start position.

5 Star jump

TIME 40sec **REST** 20sec

Stand tall with your chest up, abs engaged and hands by your sides. Jump up and bring both feet out wide to the sides while raising your arms to the sides so your hands finish above your head. Jump back from the wide stance to the start position, lowering your arms as you go.

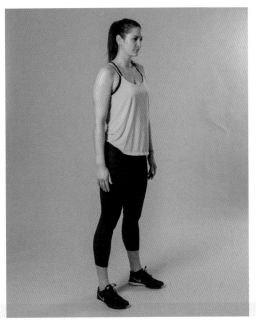
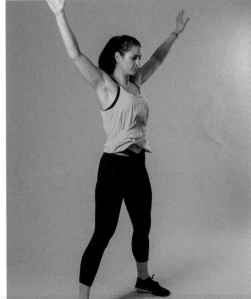

6 Speed skaters

TIME 40sec **REST** 20sec

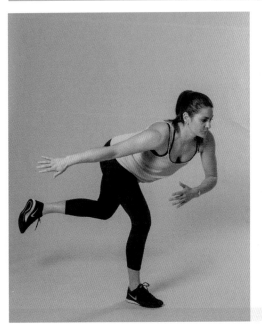
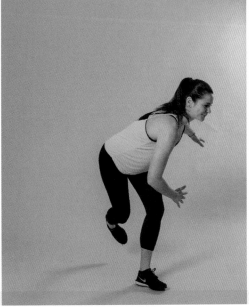

Stand tall on one leg with your chest up and abs engaged. Leap up and across to land on your other leg, swinging your arms for momentum. Your non-standing foot should go behind your standing leg. As soon as you land on your other foot leap straight back into the next rep, keeping your movements fast but controlled.

7 Rolling plank

TIME 40sec **REST** 20sec

Get onto your forearms with your elbows below your shoulders. Engage your abs, then raise your hips so that your body forms a straight line. Hold this position. Roll one side of your hips down towards the floor, then back to the top, then repeat on the other side. Continue alternating.

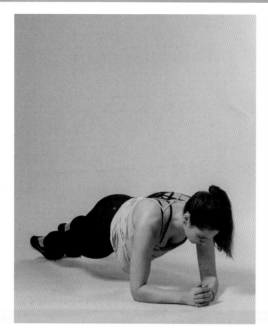 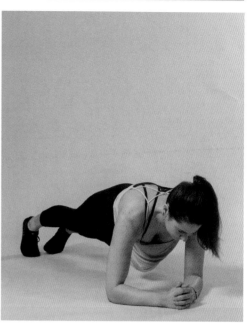

8 Lying leg raise

TIME 40sec **REST** 2min

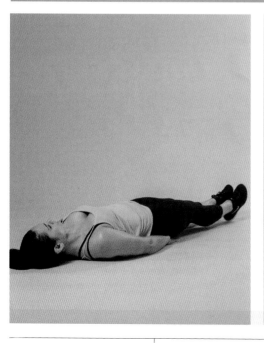 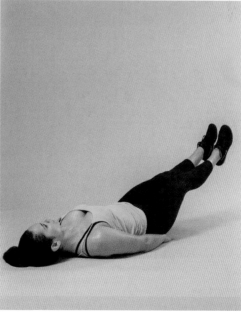

Lie flat on your back with your legs straight and hands by your sides. Engage your abs, then raise your feet up as high as you can, then slowly lower them. You can make the move harder and work your lower abs more by not allowing your heels to touch the floor between reps.

1 Sumo squat

TIME 30sec **REST** 30sec

DO 4
CIRCUITS
IN TOTAL

Stand tall with your feet double hip-width apart with your chest up, abs engaged and arms straight by your sides. Bend your knees to squat down as low as you can, either keeping your hands by your sides or raising them up to shoulder height. Push through your heels to straighten your legs and return to the start position.

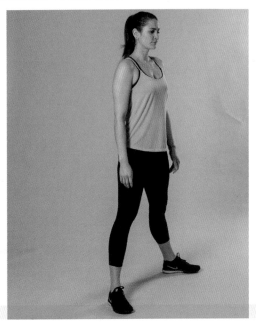
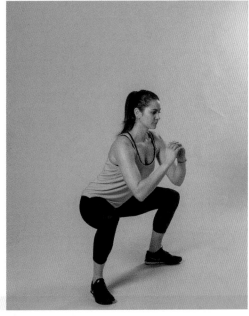

2 Chair press-up

TIME 30sec **REST** 30sec

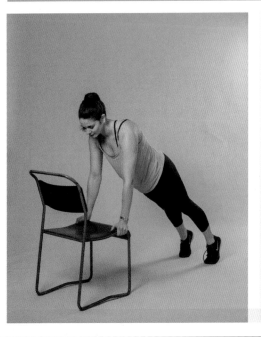
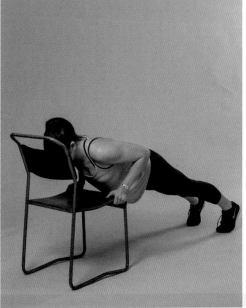

Place your hands on the seat of a chair in front of you with straight arms and your body straight from head to heels. Engage your abs and bend your elbows to lower your chest towards the seat. Go as low as you can, then press back up to straighten your arms and return to the start position.

3 Lunge

TIME 30sec **REST** 30sec

Stand tall with your chest up and abs engaged. Take a big step forwards with your left foot, then bend both knees to lunge down until your knees almost touch the floor. Push through your front foot to return to the start, then step forwards with your right foot and repeat the move. Alternate sides with each rep.

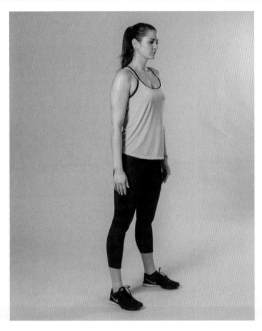
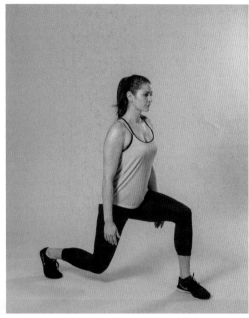

4 Glute bridge

TIME 30sec **REST** 30sec

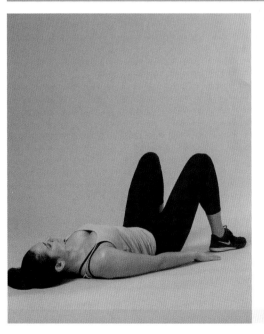
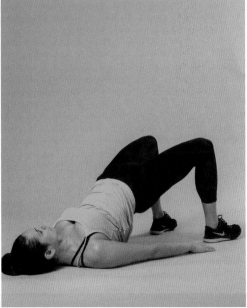

Lie flat on your back with your hands by your side and your knees bent. Engage your abs and your glutes (bum muscles), then raise your hips off the floor. Squeeze your glutes hard at the top, then lower your hips to return to the start position.

5 High knees

TIME 30sec **REST** 30sec

Stand tall with your chest up and abs engaged. Start sprinting on the spot, swinging your arms and bringing your knees up as high as possible. You can also put your arms out straight in front of you and try to make your knees hit your palms with each step.

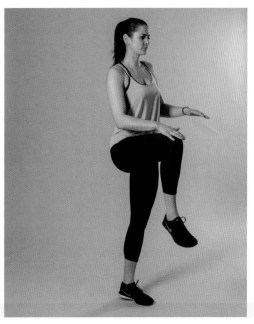
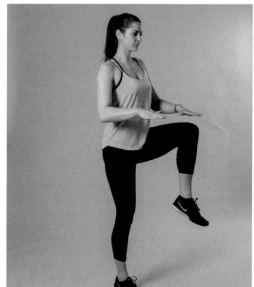

6 Butt kicks

TIME 30sec **REST** 30sec

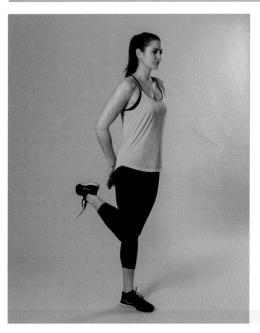
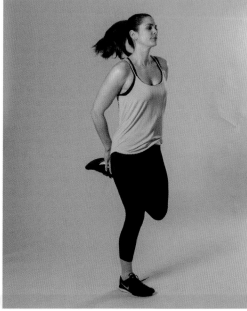

Stand tall with your chest up. Kick one foot up behind you so your heel touches your bum, then return it to the floor and kick the other foot up. Remain on the same spot, and don't move forwards or backwards. Keep each butt kick fast but controlled, with your abs engaged throughout.

7 Shoulder tap planks

TIME 30sec **REST** 30sec

Get into position with your palms on the floor and your body in a straight line. Keep your abs and glutes engaged to hold this position without letting your hips sag. Lift one hand off the floor and tap your opposite shoulder. Return it and repeat with your other hand. Keep your breathing controlled.

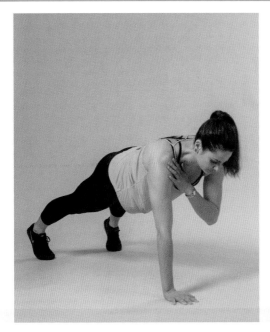
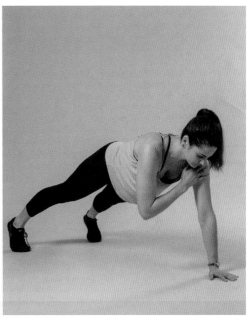

8 Mountain climber

TIME 30sec **REST** 2min

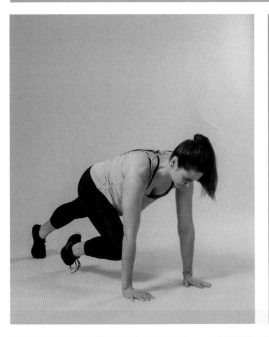
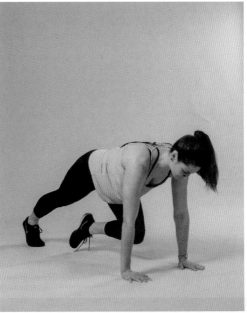

Get on all fours with your arms and legs straight. Without letting your hips sag, draw one knee up and bring it towards the elbow on the same side. Straighten that leg, then repeat, bringing your other knee towards your elbow. Keep your abs engaged throughout and keep the reps fast.

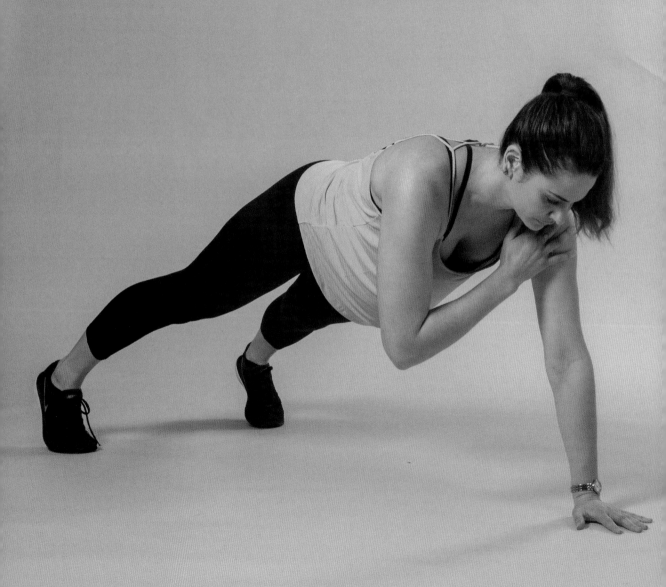

Week 2

Leave a day between each session in this, and every, week

This week you'll do the exact same sessions as in week one - but with one big change to help you build a better body faster. For each move you'll do an extra 10 seconds of work with 10 seconds less rest. This will send your heart rate soaring and get you hot and sweaty, which is exactly what it takes to sculpt a stronger and leaner physique! Stick to the moves in order and give these three sessions all you've got!

1 Squat

TIME 40sec REST 20sec

DO 4 CIRCUITS IN TOTAL

Stand tall with your chest up, abs engaged and arms straight by your sides. Bend your knees to squat down as low as you can, either keeping your hands by your sides or raising them up to shoulder height. Push through your heels to straighten your legs and return to the start position.

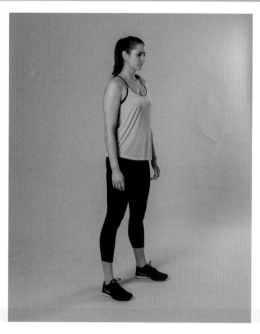
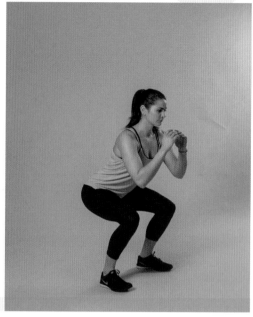

2 Chair dip - bent knees

TIME 40sec REST 20sec

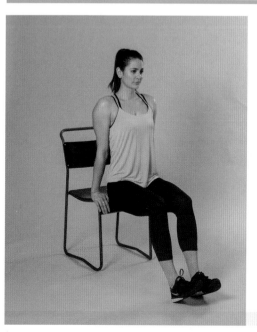
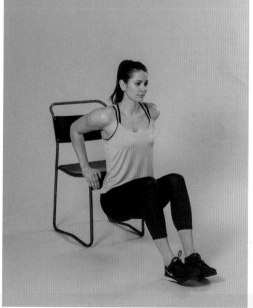

Place your hands on the edge of a chair behind you with your arms straight and knees bent. Keeping your chest up, bend your elbows to lower your bum towards the floor. Go as low as you can, then press back up to straighten your arms and return to the start position.

3 Side lunge

TIME 40sec **REST** 20sec

Stand tall with your chest up, abs engaged and arms by your sides. Take a big step to your left, then bend your left leg to lunge down. Push through your left foot to return to the start, then repeat by taking a big step to your right. Alternate sides with each rep.

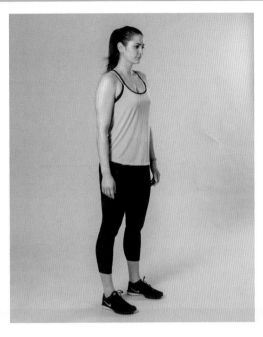
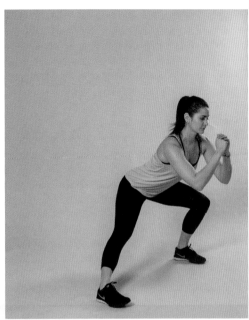

4 Alternating toe touch

TIME 40sec **REST** 20sec

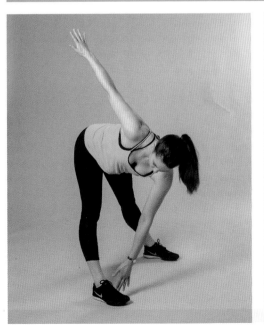
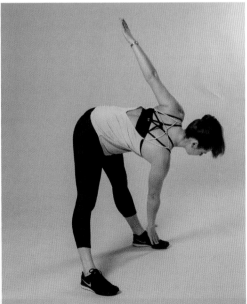

Stand tall with your chest up. Bend down from your hips, trying to keep your legs straight, and touch your right foot with your left hand. Stand back up and repeat, touching your left foot with your right hand. Alternate sides with each rep.

5 **Standing sprint**

TIME 40sec **REST** 20sec

Stand tall with your chest up and abs engaged. Sprint on the spot, raising your knees as high as possible and swinging your arms back and forth.

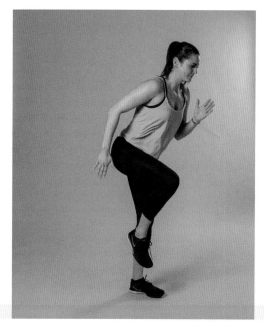
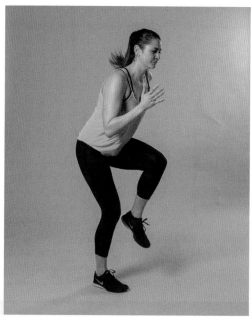

6 **Pogo**

TIME 40sec **REST** 20sec

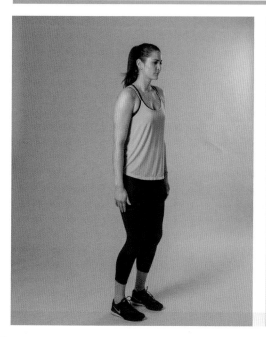
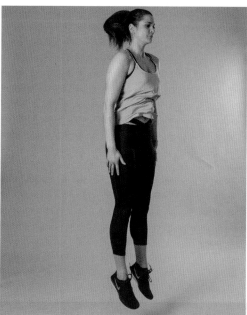

Stand tall with your chest up, abs engaged and arms by your sides. Spring straight up into the air, keeping your arms by your sides. Land on both feet and go straight into the next jump.

7 **Bicycles**

TIME 40sec **REST** 20sec

Lie on your back with your fingers by your temples and legs straight. Raise your torso up, engage your abs, and lift up your feet. Crunch up and rotate to one side, bringing your opposite knee in to touch your elbow. Reverse the move to return to the starting position and repeat alternating sides.

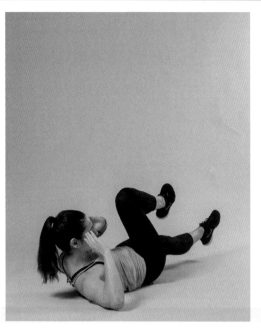
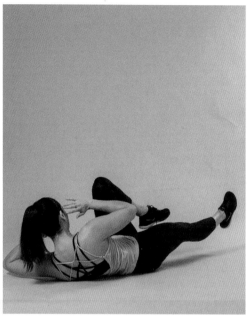

8 **Tall plank**

TIME 40sec **REST** 2min

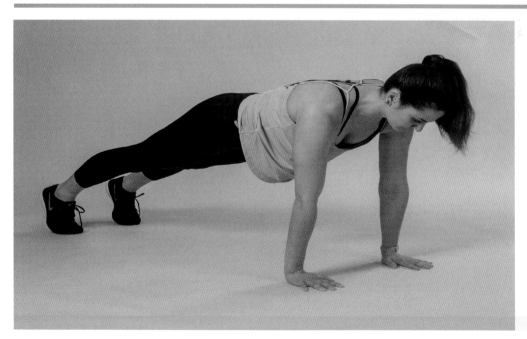

Get into position with your palms on the floor, your wrists underneath your shoulders and your body in a straight line from head to heels. Keep your abs and glutes (bum muscles) engaged to hold this position without letting your hips sag. Keep your breathing controlled and relaxed.

1 Prisoner squat

TIME 50sec **REST** 10sec

DO 4
CIRCUITS
IN TOTAL

Stand tall with your chest up, abs engaged and elbows bent with your hands behind your head Bend your knees to squat down as low as you can. Push through your heels to straighten your legs and return to the start position.

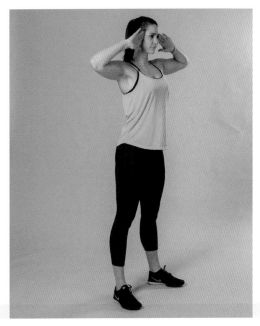
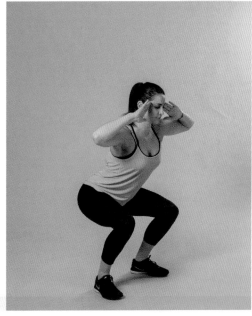

2 Knee press-up

TIME 50sec **REST** 10sec

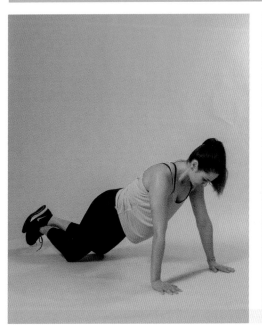
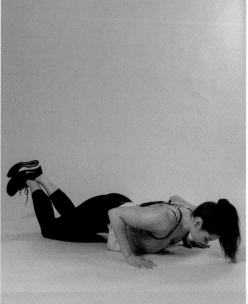

Get on your hands and knees with your bodyweight shifted forwards. Engage your abs and bend your elbows to lower your chest towards the floor. Go as low as you can, then press back up to straighten your arms and return to the start position.

3 Curtsy lunge

TIME 50sec **REST** 10sec

Stand tall with your chest up, your abs engaged and your hands by your sides. Keeping your chest up place one foot behind the other, then bend both knees to lunge down until your back knee almost touches the floor. Push off your rear foot to return to the start position, then repeat, leading with your other leg.

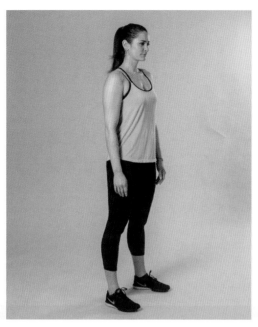
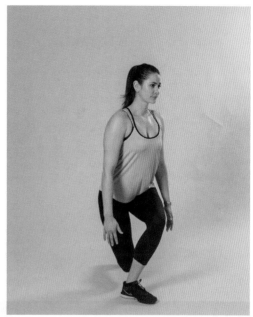

4 RDL

TIME 50sec **REST** 10sec

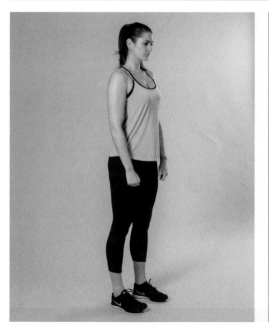
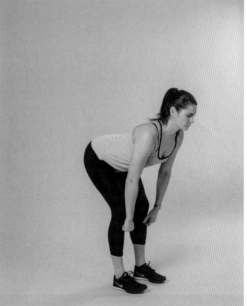

Stand tall with your chest up and abs engaged. With a slight bend in your knees, bend forwards from the hips and reach down the front of your legs, touching your fingertips to them as low down as possible. Stand up to return to the start position.

5 **Star jump**

TIME 50sec **REST** 10sec

Stand tall with your chest up, abs engaged and hands by your sides. Jump up and bring both feet out wide to the sides while raising your arms to the sides so your hands finish above your head. Jump back from the wide stance to the start position, lowering your arms as you go.

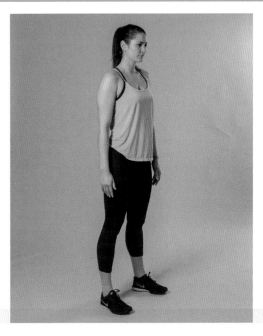
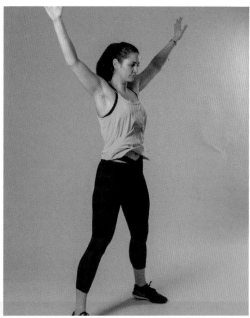

6 **Speed skaters**

TIME 50sec **REST** 10sec

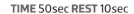

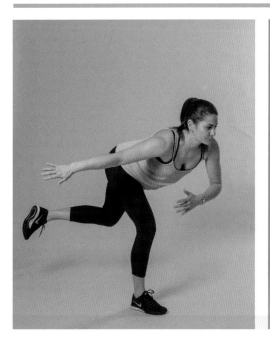
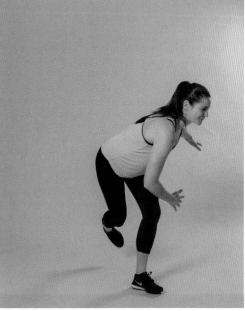

Stand tall on one leg with your chest up and abs engaged. Leap up and across to land on your other leg, swinging your arms for momentum. Your non-standing foot should go behind your standing leg. As soon as you land on your other foot leap straight back into the next rep, keeping your movements fast but controlled.

7 Rolling plank

TIME 50sec **REST** 10sec

Get onto your forearms with your elbows below your shoulders. Engage your abs, then raise your hips so that your body forms a straight line. Hold this position. Roll one side of your hips down towards the floor, then back to the top, then repeat on the other side. Continue alternating.

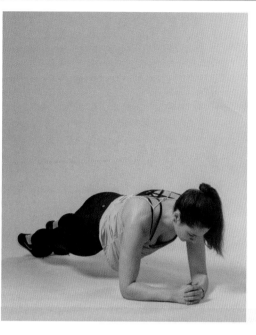
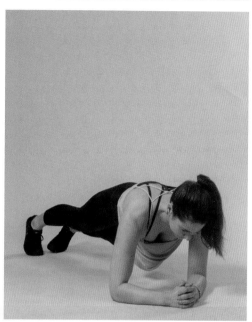

8 Lying leg raise

TIME 50sec **REST** 2min

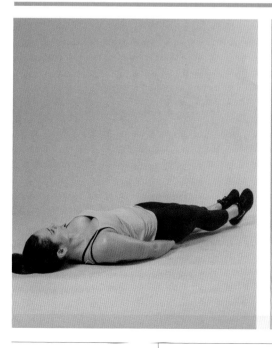
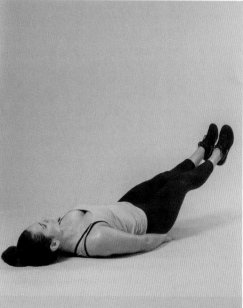

Lie flat on your back with your legs straight and hands by your sides. Engage your abs, then raise your feet up as high as you can, then slowly lower them. You can make the move harder and work your lower abs more by not allowing your heels to touch the floor between reps.

1 Sumo squat

TIME 40sec **REST** 20sec

DO 4 CIRCUITS IN TOTAL

Stand tall with your feet double hip-width apart with your chest up, abs engaged and arms straight by your sides. Bend your knees to squat down as low as you can, either keeping your hands by your sides or raising them up to shoulder height. Push through your heels to straighten your legs and return to the start position.

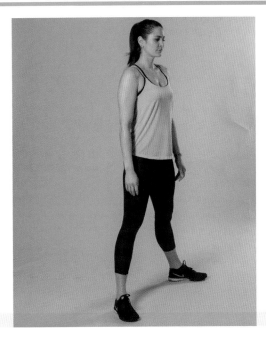
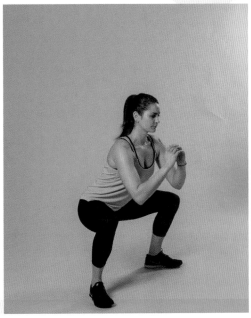

2 Chair press-up

TIME 40sec **REST** 20sec

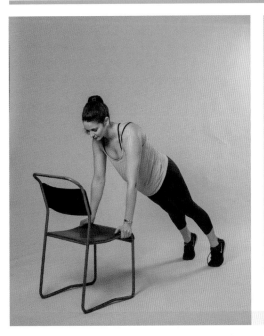
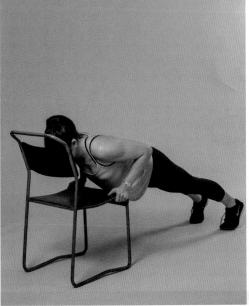

Place your hands on the seat of a chair in front of you with straight arms and your body straight from head to heels. Engage your abs and bend your elbows to lower your chest towards the seat. Go as low as you can, then press back up to straighten your arms and return to the start position.

3 **Lunge**

TIME 40sec **REST** 20sec

Stand tall with your chest up and abs engaged. Take a big step forwards with your left foot, then bend both knees to lunge down until your knees almost touch the floor. Push through your front foot to return to the start, then step forwards with your right foot and repeat the move. Alternate sides with each rep.

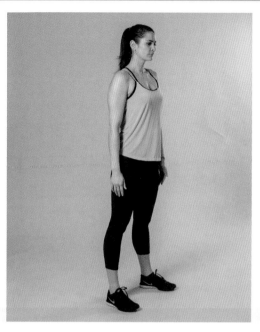
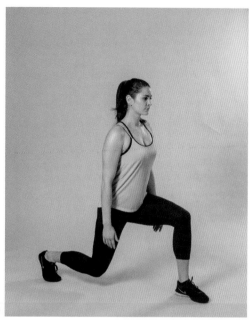

4 **Glute bridge**

TIME 40sec **REST** 20sec

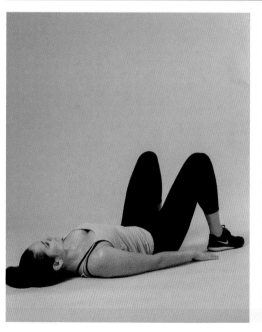
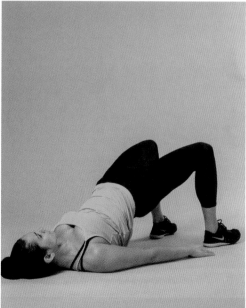

Lie flat on your back with your hands by your side and your knees bent. Engage your abs and your glutes (bum muscles), then raise your hips off the floor. Squeeze your glutes hard at the top, then lower your hips to return to the start position.

5 High knees

TIME 40sec REST 20sec

Stand tall with your chest up and abs engaged. Start sprinting on the spot, swinging your arms and bringing your knees up as high as possible. You can also put your arms out straight in front of you and try to make your knees hit your palms with each step.

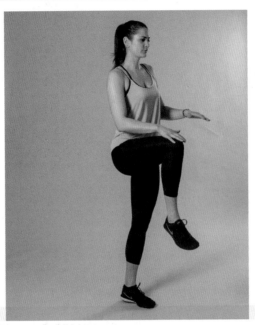
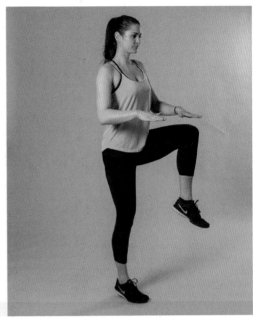

6 Butt kicks

TIME 40sec REST 20sec

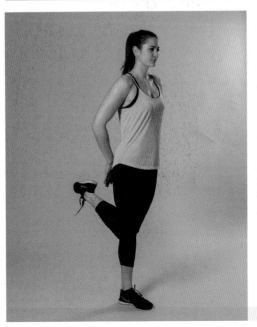
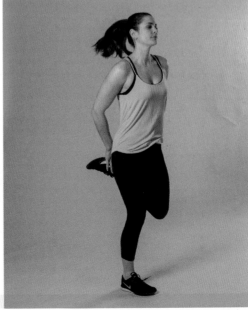

Stand tall with your chest up. Kick one foot up behind you so your heel touches your bum, then return it to the floor and kick the other foot up. Remain on the same spot, and don't move forwards or backwards. Keep each butt kick fast but controlled, with your abs engaged throughout.

7 Shoulder tap planks

TIME 40sec **REST** 20sec

Get into position with your palms on the floor and your body in a straight line. Keep your abs and glutes engaged to hold this position without letting your hips sag. Lift one hand off the floor and tap your opposite shoulder. Return it and repeat with your other hand. Keep your breathing controlled.

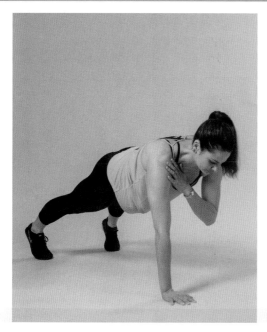
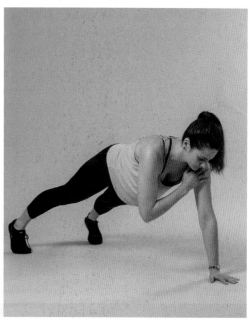

8 Mountain climber

TIME 40sec **REST** 2min

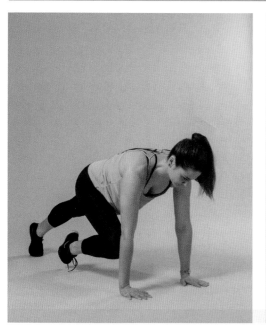
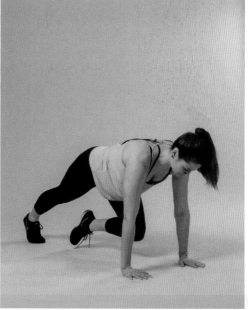

Get on all fours with your arms and legs straight. Without letting your hips sag, draw one knee up and bring it towards the elbow on the same side. Straighten that leg, then repeat, bringing your other knee towards your elbow. Keep your abs engaged throughout and keep the reps fast.

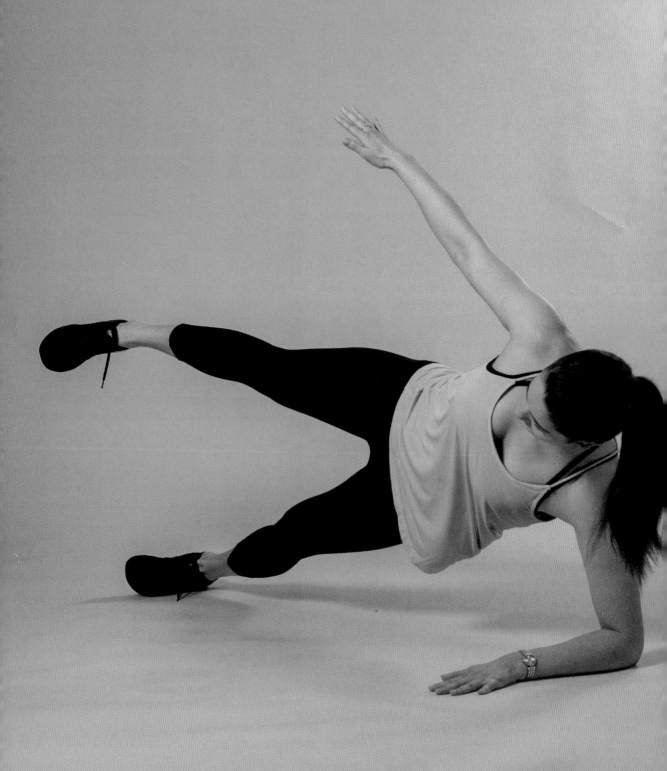

Week 3

Leave a day between each session in this, and every, week

For the final fortnight of this four-week plan we've changed all the exercises to work your heart, lungs and muscles in new and challenging ways to help your burn off as much body fat as possible while also toning and defining your muscles. There's still three eight-move total-body sessions, so follow the order and the work and rest durations detailed to keep your better-body mission well on track!

1 Overhead squat

TIME 30sec **REST** 30sec

DO 4 CIRCUITS IN TOTAL

Stand tall with your chest up, abs engaged and arms raised directly overhead. Bend your knees to squat down as low as you can, keeping your arms straight overhead. Push through your heels to straighten your legs and return to the start position.

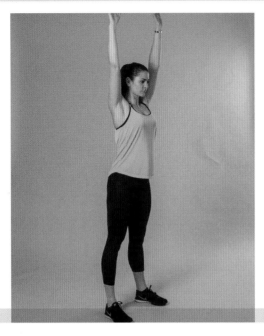
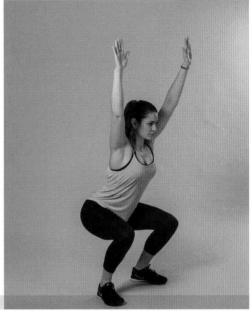

2 Sumo squat

TIME 30sec **REST** 30sec

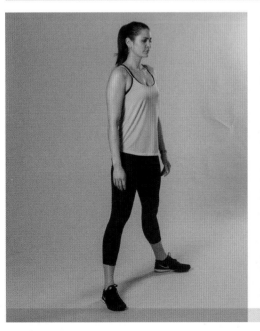
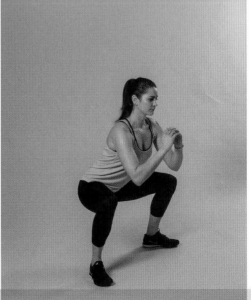

Stand tall with your feet double hip–width apart with your chest up, abs engaged and arms straight by your sides. Bend your knees to squat down as low as you can, either keeping your hands by your sides or raising them up to shoulder height. Push through your heels to straighten your legs.

3 Chair dip - straight legs

TIME 30sec REST 30sec

Place your hands on the edge of a chair behind you with your arms straight and legs straight. Keeping your chest up, bend your elbows to lower your bum towards the floor. Go as low as you can, then press back up to straighten your arms and return to the start position.

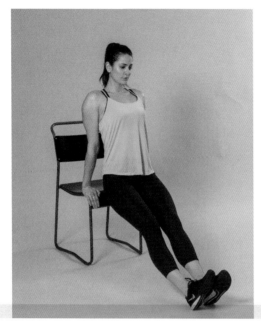
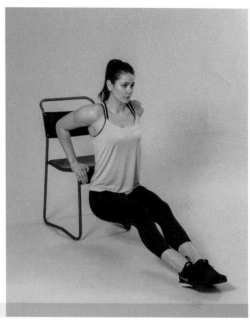

4 Prisoner lunge

TIME 30sec REST 30sec

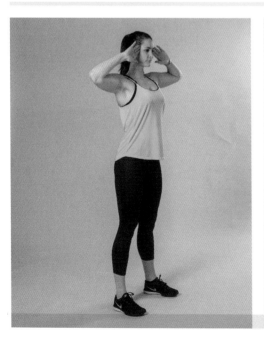
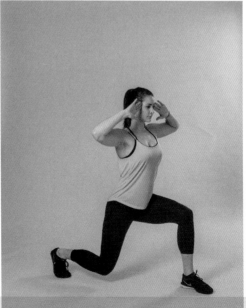

Stand tall with your fingers by your temples. Take a big step forwards with your right foot, then bend both knees to lunge down until your knees almost touch the floor. Push through your front foot to return to the start, then step forwards with your left foot and repeat the move. Alternate sides with each rep.

5 Burpee

TIME 30sec REST 30sec

Stand tall with your arms by your sides. Drop down so your palms are on the floor with your knees by your chest. Kick your legs out so your body forms a straight line from head to heels. Bring your knees back under your body, then jump up into the air. As you land, go straight into the next rep.

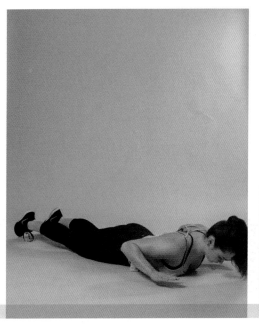
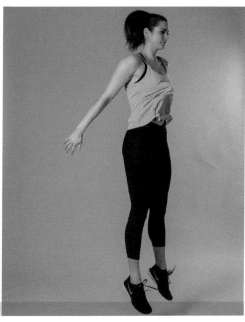

6 Crunch

TIME 30sec REST 30sec

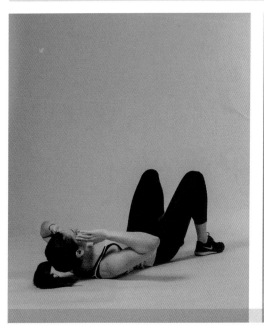
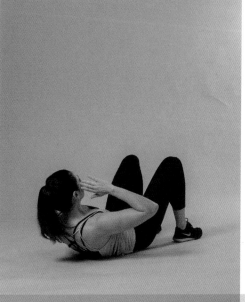

Lie flat on your back with your knees bent and feet flat on the floor, and bend your arms so your fingers touch the side of your head. Engage your abs, then raise your torso off the floor without tensing your neck. Keep that tension on your abs as you slowly lower your torso back to the floor.

7 Heel taps

TIME 30sec **REST** 30sec

Stand tall. Keeping your arms straight, engage your abs and reach down with your right hand to tap your left heel, then your right hand to tap your left heel. Keep alternating. Keep your breathing controlled and relaxed.

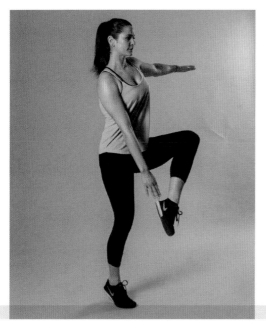
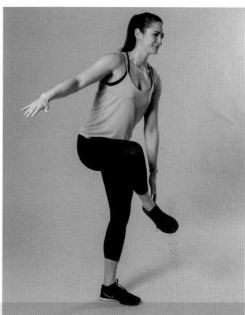

8 Side plank

TIME 30sec **REST** 2min

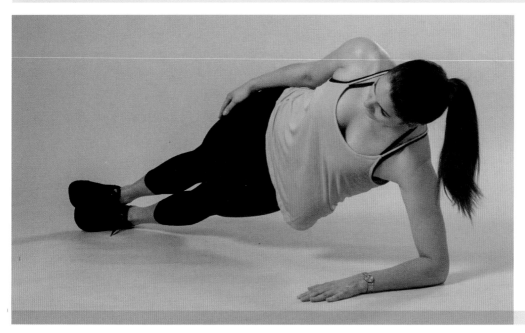

Lie on one side, supporting your upper body on that forearm. Engage your abs, then raise your hips so that your body forms a straight line. Keep your abs and glutes engaged to hold this position without letting your hips sag. Keep your breathing controlled. Halfway through switch sides.

1 Split squat - left

TIME 40sec **REST** 20sec

DO 4 CIRCUITS IN TOTAL

Stand tall with your left foot forward and your chest up and abs engaged. Bend both knees until your right knee almost touches the floor. Push through your front foot to return to the start and repeat.

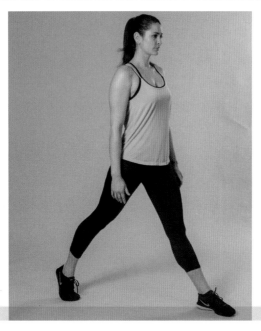
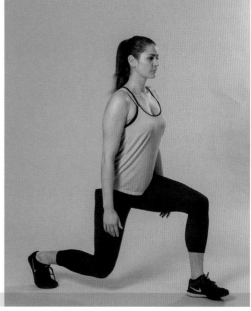

2 Split squat - right

TIME 40sec **REST** 20sec

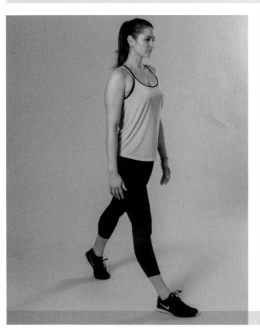
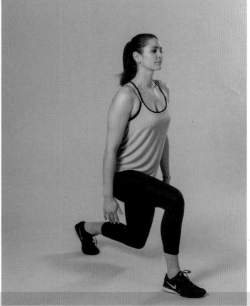

Stand tall with your right foot forward and your chest up and abs engaged. Bend both knees until your left knee almost touches the floor. Push through your front foot to return to the start and repeat.

3 **Press-up**

Get on all fours with your legs and arms straight, your hands under your shoulders and your body in a straight line from head to heels. Engage your abs and bend your elbows to lower your chest towards the floor. Go as low as you can, then press back up to straighten your arms and return to the start position.

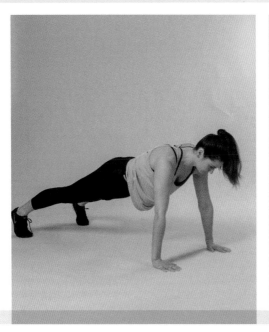
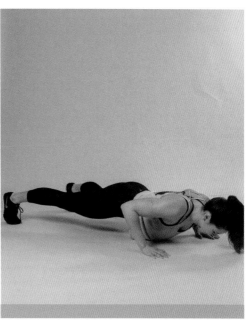

4 **Curtsy lunge**

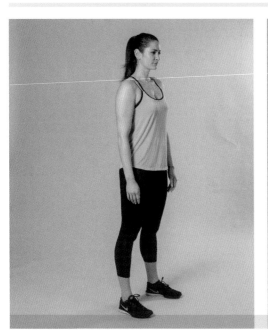
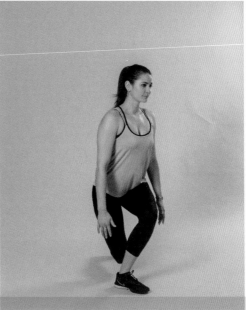

Stand tall with your chest up and hands by your sides. Place one foot behind the other, then bend both knees to lunge down until your back knee almost touches the floor. Push off your rear foot to return to the start position, then repeat, leading with your other leg. Alternate legs with each rep.

5 **Squat jump**

TIME 40sec **REST** 20sec

Stand tall with your chest up, abs engaged and arms straight by your sides. Bend your knees to squat down as low as you can, and swing your arms backwards. Push through your heels to straighten your legs and jump powerfully off the floor. Land on both feet and go straight into the next rep.

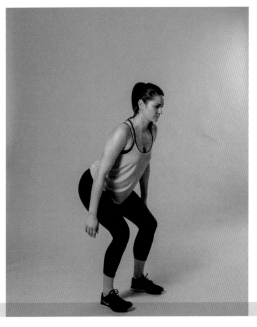
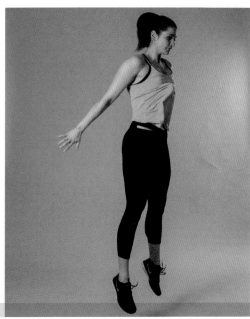

6 **Reverse crunch**

TIME 40sec **REST** 20sec

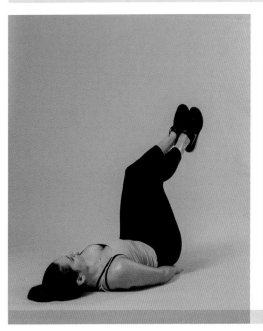
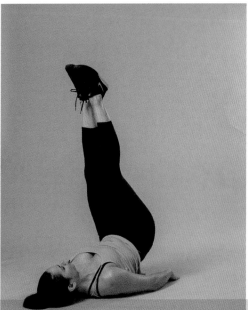

Lie flat on your back with your arms flat on the floor and knees bent. Use your lower abs to draw your knees in towards your chest, then raise your hips up off the ground, then lower back to the start, keeping your abs fully engaged throughout.

7 **Seated Russian twist**

TIME 40sec **REST** 20sec

Sit up with your chest up, abs engaged and a slight bend in your knees. Use your abs to rotate your torso to one side, then return to the middle and rotate to the other side. Make the move harder by raising your heels off the floor and keeping them raised.

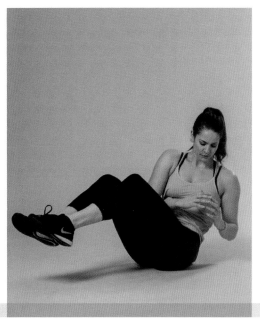
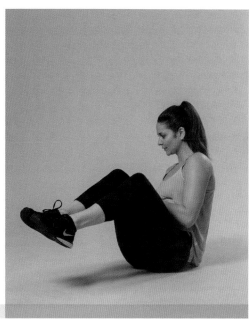

8 **Plank**

TIME 40sec **REST** 2min

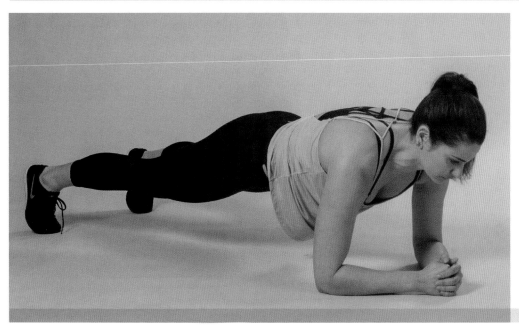

Get into position on your forearms with your elbows underneath your shoulders. Engage your abs, then raise your hips so that your body forms a straight line. Hold this position by keeping your abs and glutes engaged to stop your hips sagging. Keep your breathing controlled and relaxed.

1 Prisoner squat

TIME 30sec **REST** 30sec

DO 4 CIRCUITS IN TOTAL

Stand tall with your chest up, abs engaged and elbows bent with your fingers by your temples. Bend your knees to squat down as low as you can. Push through your heels to straighten your legs and return to the start position.

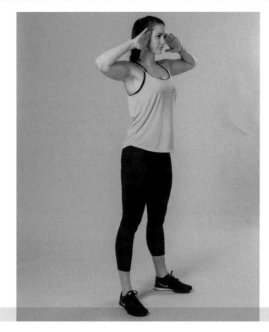
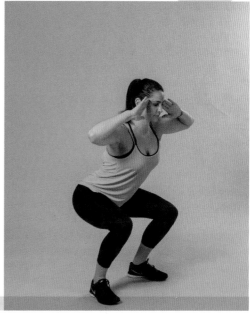

2 Pulse squat

TIME 30sec **REST** 30sec

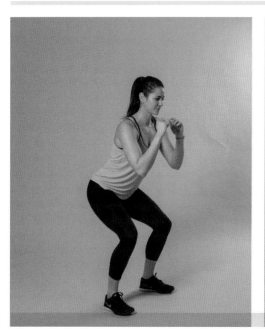
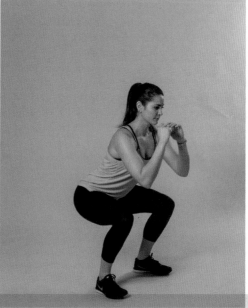

Stand tall then bend your knees to squat down as low as you can, either keeping your arms by your sides or raising them to shoulder height. In the bottom position of the squat, "pulse" up and down three times, then straighten your legs to return to the start position.

3 Diamond knee press-up

TIME 30sec REST 30sec

Placing your hands close together so your thumbs and index fingers touch, lower your torso until your chest is just above the floor then press back up to get back to the start and repeat the move.

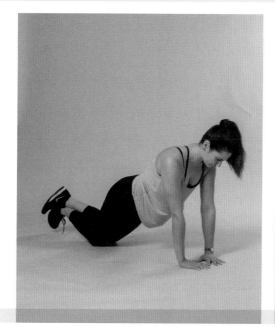
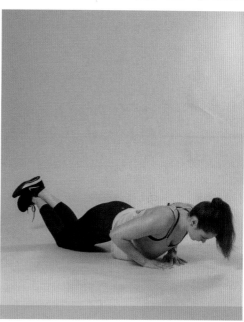

4 Reverse lunge

TIME 30sec REST 30sec

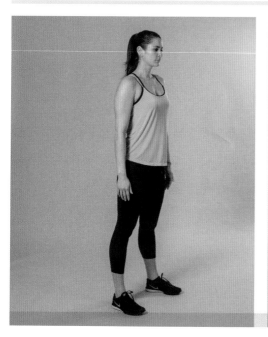
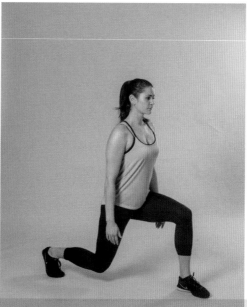

Stand tall with your chest up. Take a big step backwards with your right foot, then bend both knees to lunge down until your knee almost touches the floor. Push through your back foot to return to the start, then step backwards with your left foot and repeat the move. Alternate sides with each rep.

5 Plank jack

TIME 30sec **REST** 30sec

Get into position, supporting yourself on your forearms with your elbows underneath your shoulders. Engage your abs, then raise your hips so that your body forms a straight line from head to heels. Without letting your hips sag, jump both feet out to the sides, then back in and repeat.

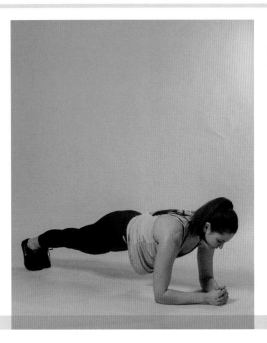 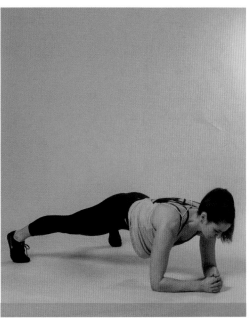

6 Crunch reach

TIME 30sec **REST** 30sec

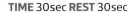

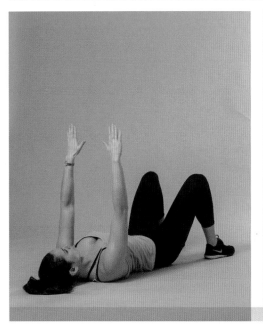 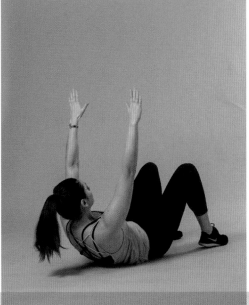

Lie flat on your back with your knees bent and your arms straight. Crunch upward, reaching your hands as high up as possible. Pause at the top of the movement, then lower back to the start.

7 Plank toe taps

TIME 30sec **REST** 30sec

Get into position and engage your abs, then raise your hips so that your body forms a straight line from head to heels. Without letting your hips sag, lift and move one foot out as far as you can to the side. Tap your toe down on the floor then bring it back in and repeat with the other foot.

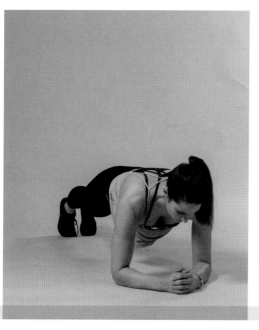
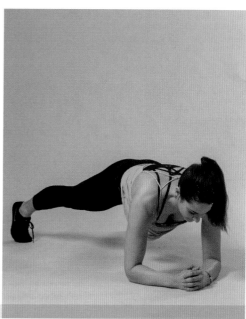

8 Side plank star

TIME 30sec **REST** 2min

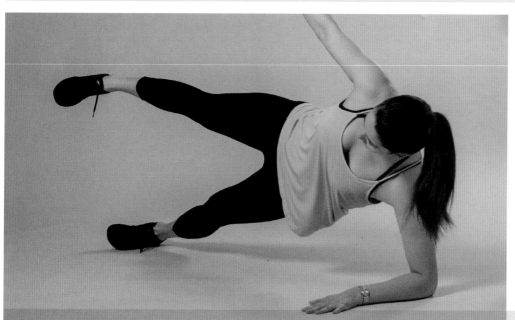

Lie on one side, supporting your upper body on that forearm. Engage your abs, then raise your hips so that your body forms a straight line. From there raise your top arm and leg up into the air and hold this position, swapping sides halfway through the work period.

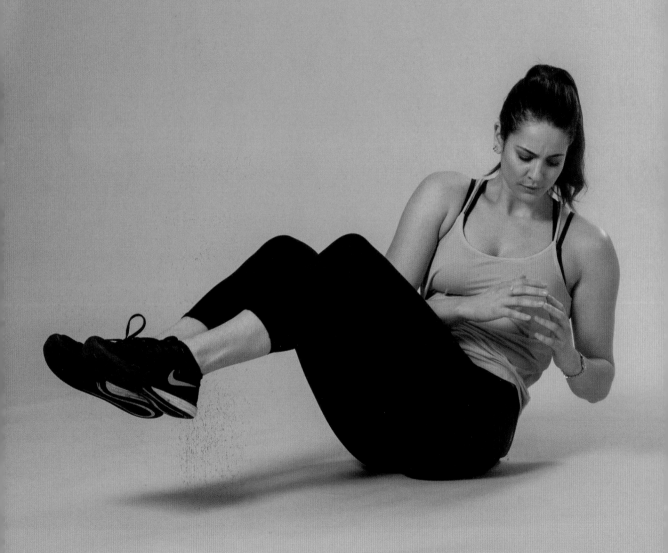

Week 4

Leave a day
between
each session
in this, and
every, week

In this final week of the plan the exercises are the same and in the same order as last week, but again we've increased the duration of the work periods by 10 seconds - and reduced each rest period by the same amount of time - to push your body even harder to keep the positive body composition changes coming so you finish this first plan stronger, leaner and healthier than ever before. Let's do this!

1 Overhead squat

TIME 40sec **REST** 20sec

DO 4
CIRCUITS
IN TOTAL

Stand tall with your chest up, abs engaged and arms raised directly overhead. Bend your knees to squat down as low as you can, keeping your arms straight overhead. Push through your heels to straighten your legs and return to the start position.

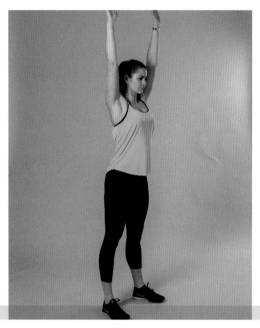
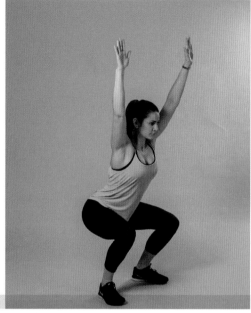

2 Sumo squat

TIME 40sec **REST** 20sec

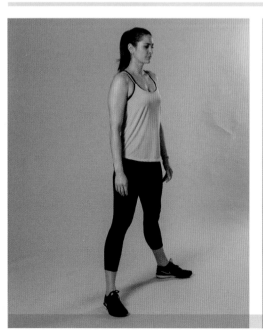
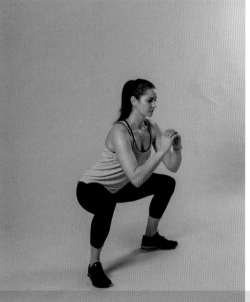

Stand tall with your feet double hip–width apart with your chest up, abs engaged and arms straight by your sides. Bend your knees to squat down as low as you can, either keeping your hands by your sides or raising them up to shoulder height. Push through your heels to straighten your legs.

3 Chair dip - straight legs

TIME 40sec **REST** 20sec

Place your hands on the edge of a chair behind you with your arms straight and legs straight. Keeping your chest up, bend your elbows to lower your bum towards the floor. Go as low as you can, then press back up to straighten your arms and return to the start position.

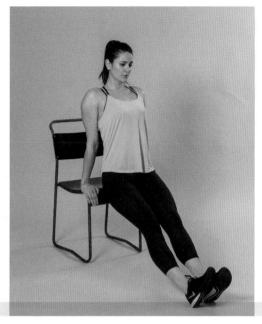
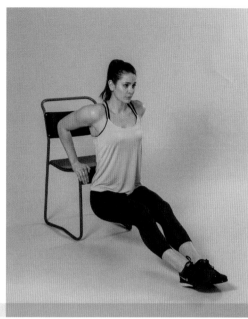

4 Prisoner lunge

TIME 40sec **REST** 20sec

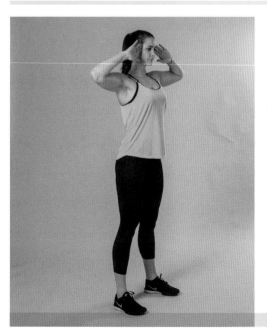
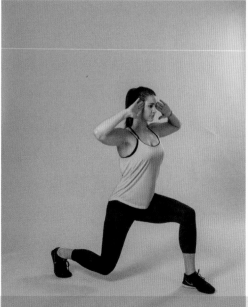

Stand tall with your fingers by your temples. Take a big step forwards with your right foot, then bend both knees to lunge down until your knees almost touch the floor. Push through your front foot to return to the start, then step forwards with your left foot and repeat the move. Alternate sides with each rep.

5 Burpee

TIME 40sec **REST** 20sec

Stand tall with your arms by your sides. Drop down so your palms are on the floor with your knees by your chest. Kick your legs out so your body forms a straight line from head to heels. Bring your knees back under your body, then jump up into the air. As you land, go straight into the next rep.

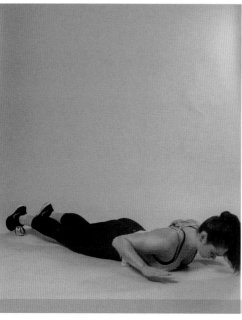
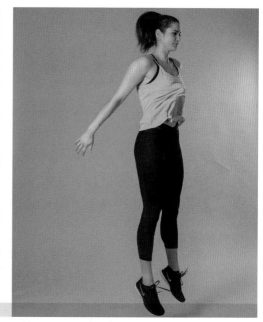

6 Crunch

TIME 40sec **REST** 20sec

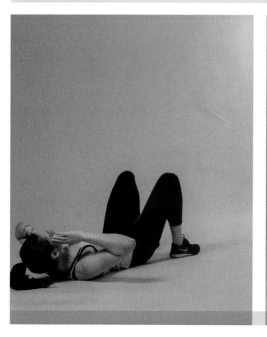
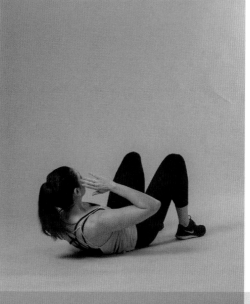

Lie flat on your back with your knees bent and feet flat on the floor, and bend your arms so your fingers touch the side of your head. Engage your abs, then raise your torso off the floor without tensing your neck. Keep that tension on your abs as you slowly lower your torso back to the floor.

7 **Heel taps**

TIME 40sec REST 20sec

Stand tall. Keeping your arms straight, engage your abs and reach down with your left hand to tap your right heel, then your right hand to tap your left heel. Keep alternating. Keep your breathing controlled and relaxed.

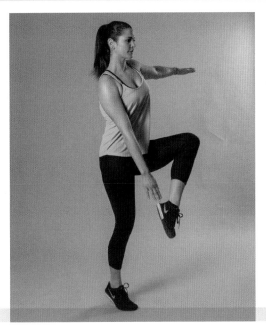
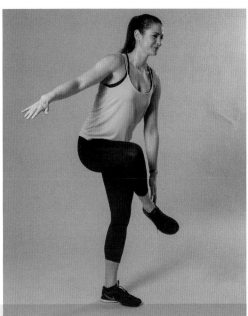

8 **Side plank**

TIME 40sec REST 2min

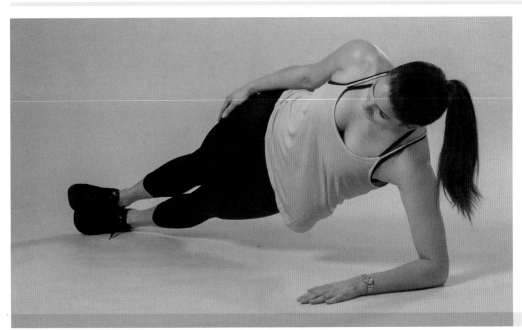

Lie on one side, supporting your upper body on that forearm. Engage your abs, then raise your hips so that your body forms a straight line. Keep your abs and glutes engaged to hold this position without letting your hips sag. Keep your breathing controlled and halfway through switch sides.

1 Split squat - left

TIME 50sec **REST** 10sec

DO 4 CIRCUITS IN TOTAL

Stand tall with your left foot forward and your chest up and abs engaged. Bend both knees until your right knee almost touches the floor. Push through your front foot to return to the start and repeat.

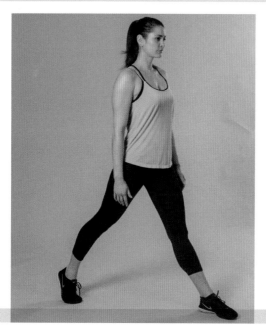
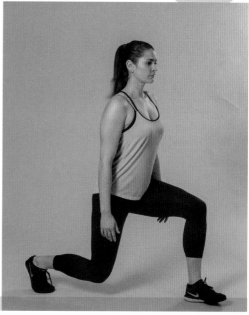

2 Split squat - right

TIME 50sec **REST** 10sec

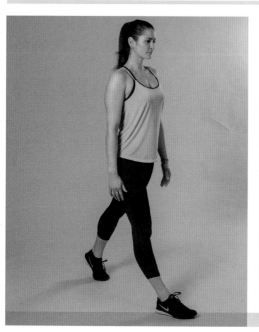
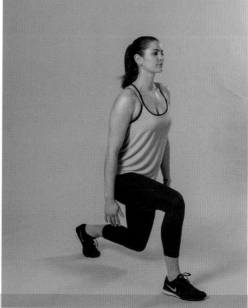

Stand tall with your right foot forward and your chest up and abs engaged. Bend both knees until your left knee almost touches the floor. Push through your front foot to return to the start and repeat.

3 Press-up

TIME 50sec **REST** 10sec

Get on all fours with your legs and arms straight, your hands under your shoulders and your body in a straight line from head to heels. Engage your abs and bend your elbows to lower your chest towards the floor. Go as low as you can, then press back up to straighten your arms and return to the start position.

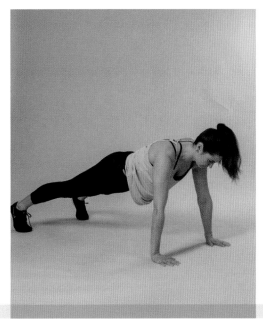
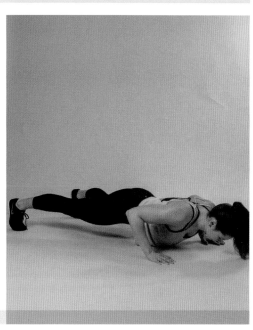

4 Curtsy lunge

TIME 50sec **REST** 10sec

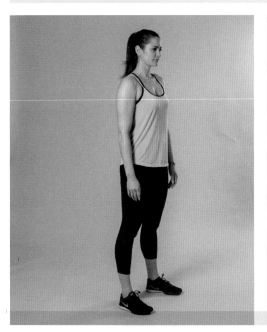
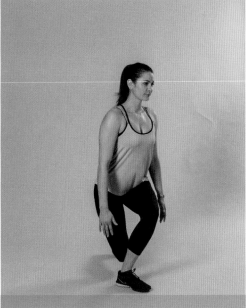

Stand tall with your chest up and hands by your sides. Place one foot behind the other, then bend both knees to lunge down until your back knee almost touches the floor. Push off your rear foot to return to the start position, then repeat, leading with your other leg. Alternate legs with each rep.

5 **Squat jump**

TIME 50sec **REST** 10sec

Stand tall with your chest up, abs engaged and arms straight by your sides. Bend your knees to squat down as low as you can, and swing your arms backwards. Push through your heels to straighten your legs and jump powerfully off the floor. Land on both feet and go straight into the next rep.

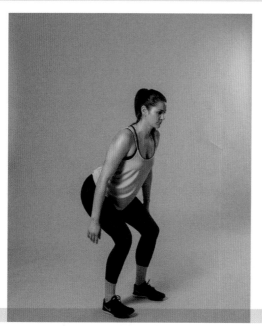
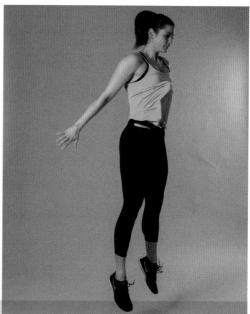

6 **Reverse crunch**

TIME 50sec **REST** 10sec

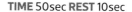
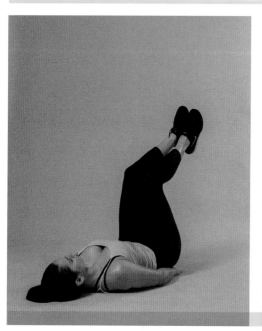
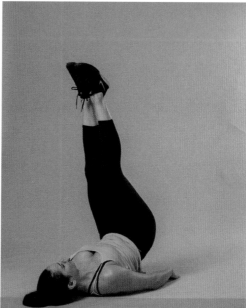

Lie flat on your back with your arms flat on the floor and knees bent. Use your lower abs to draw your knees in towards your chest, then raise your hips up off the ground, then lower back to the start, keeping your abs fully engaged throughout.

7 Seated Russian twist

TIME 50sec REST 10sec

Sit up with your chest up, abs engaged and a slight bend in your knees. Use your abs to rotate your torso to one side, then return to the middle and rotate to the other side. Make the move harder by raising your heels off the floor and keeping them raised.

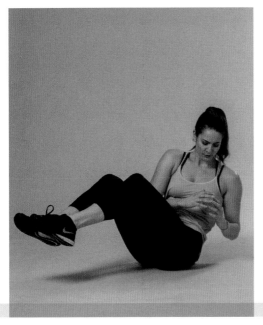 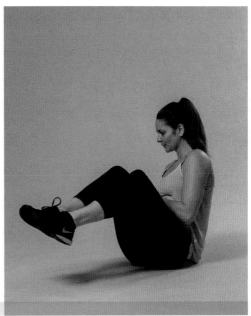

8 Plank

TIME 50sec REST 2min

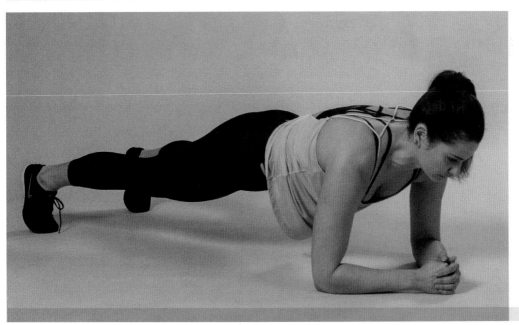

Get into position on your forearms with your elbows underneath your shoulders. Engage your abs, then raise your hips so that your body forms a straight line. Hold this position by keeping your abs and glutes engaged to stop your hips sagging. Keep your breathing controlled and relaxed.

1 Prisoner squat

TIME 40sec **REST** 20sec

DO 4 CIRCUITS IN TOTAL

Stand tall with your chest up, abs engaged and elbows bent with your hands behind your head Bend your knees to squat down as low as you can. Push through your heels to straighten your legs and return to the start position.

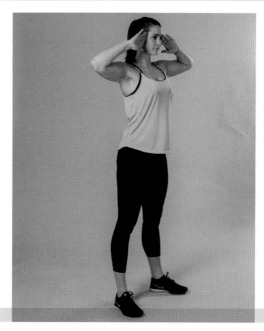
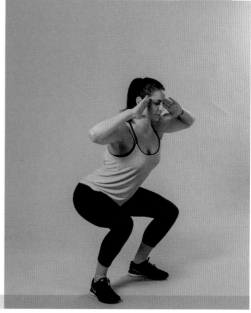

2 Pulse squat

TIME 40sec **REST** 20sec

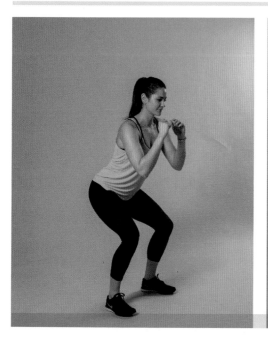
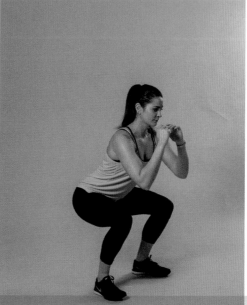

Stand tall then bend your knees to squat down as low as you can, either keeping your hands by your sides or raising them to shoulder height. In the bottom position of the squat, "pulse" up and down three times, then straighten your legs to return to the start position.

3 Diamond knee press-up

TIME 40sec **REST** 20sec

Placing your hands close together so your thumbs and index fingers touch, lower your torso until your chest is just above the floor then press back up to get back to the start and repeat the move.

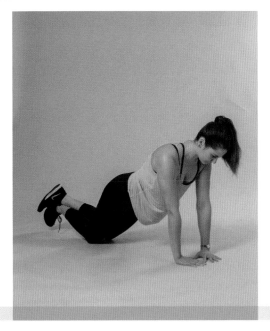
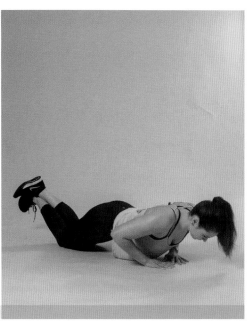

4 Reverse lunge

TIME 40sec **REST** 20sec

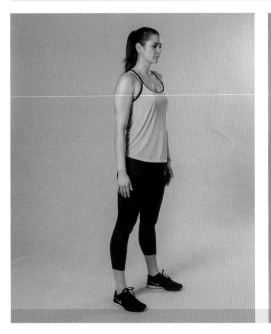
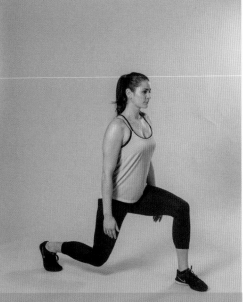

Stand tall with your chest up. Take a big step backwards with your right foot, then bend both knees to lunge down until your knees almost touch the floor. Push through your back foot to return to the start, then step backwards with your left foot and repeat the move. Alternate sides with each rep.

5 Plank jack

TIME 40sec **REST** 20sec

Get into position, supporting yourself on your forearms with your elbows underneath your shoulders. Engage your abs, then raise your hips so that your body forms a straight line from head to heels. Without letting your hips sag, jump both feet out to the sides, then back in and repeat.

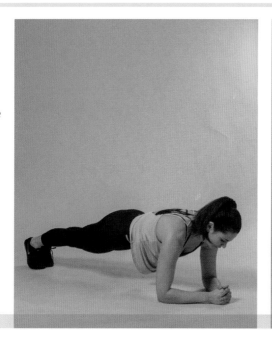
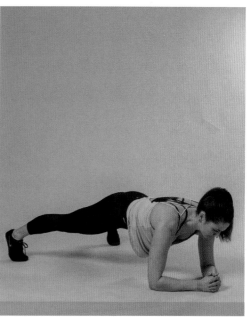

6 Crunch reach

TIME 40sec **REST** 20sec

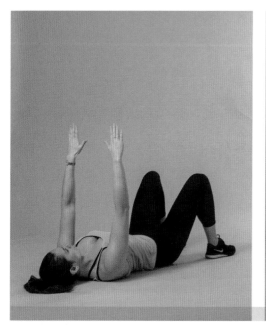
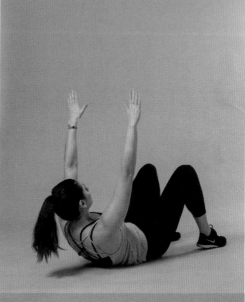

Lie flat on your back with your knees bent and your arms straight. Crunch upward, reaching your hands as high up as possible. Pause at the top of the movement, then lower back to the start.

7 Plank toe taps

TIME 40sec **REST** 20sec

Get into position and engage your abs, then raise your hips so that your body forms a straight line from head to heels. Without letting your hips sag, lift and move one foot out as far as you can to the side. Tap your toe down on the floor then bring it back in and repeat with the other foot.

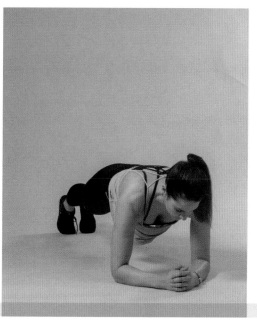
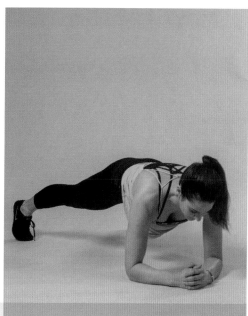

8 Side plank star

TIME 40sec **REST** 2min

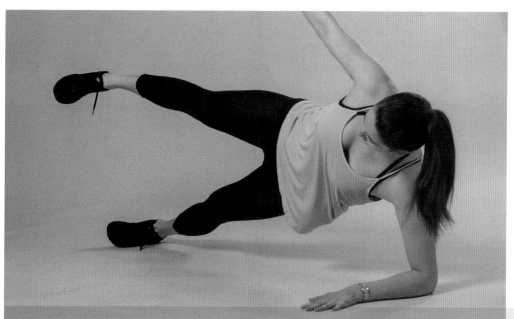

Lie on one side, supporting your upper body on that forearm. Engage your abs, then raise your hips so that your body forms a straight line. From there raise your top arm and leg up into the air and hold this position, swapping sides halfway through the work period.

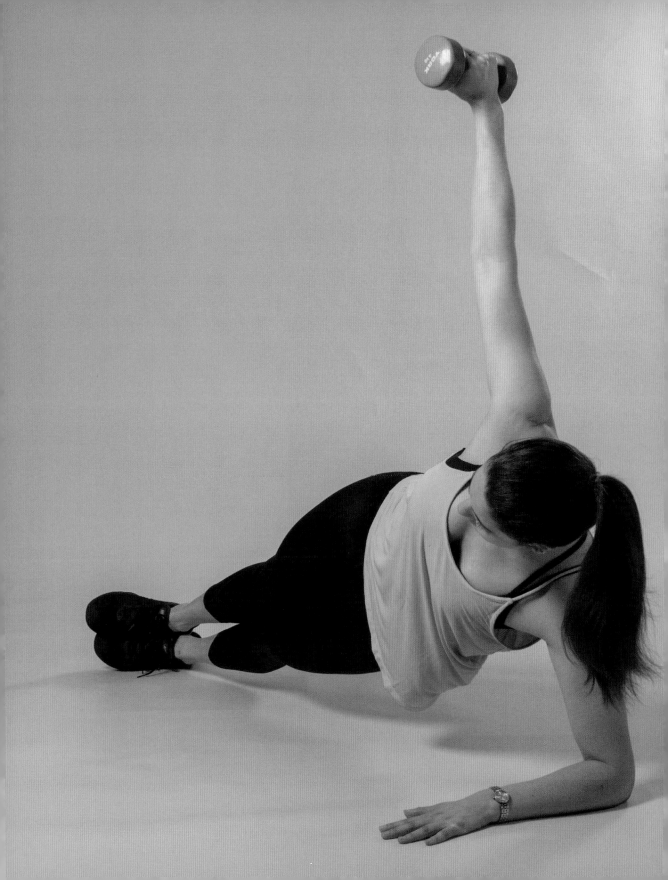

Continue your better body journey!

Congratulations on having completed your own Four-Week Bikini Body plan! Now that you're the proud owner of a leaner, stronger and fitter body, we've designed an advanced four-week training plan that includes many new moves - including dumbbell exercises - to help you continue to build a healthier body so that you look and feel great all-year long!

Workout FAQ

Q
HOW DOES THIS PLAN WORK?

A

This advanced month-long plan is very similar to the Four-Week Bikini Body plan you've already completed. There are three sessions per week – and it's important to still leave one day between doing a workout – and each one has eight different exercises to work all your major muscle groups. The one major difference is that the types of exercises are more difficult because many of them use dumbbells to increase the amount of weight your muscles must move and manage.

Q
WHY DO I NEED DUMBBELLS?

A

After four weeks of bodyweight-only exercises you will have become much stronger and fitter and therefore easily able to perform bodyweight exercises for a high amount of reps or time. To keep your positive results coming, you must make your muscles do more work than they are used to, and in this instance that means increasing the amount of resistance per exercise by holding some dumbbells. Don't worry if you've never used weights before – every new move is clearly explained.

Q
WHAT WEIGHT SHOULD I USE?

A

If you have never lifted weights before, or are coming back to this type of training after a long absence, you should start these workouts with a very light pair of dumbbells, such as 1kg or 2kg. Starting light will allow you to fully master the new movement patterns and get your muscles used to handling the additional load without a heightened risk of injury or disappointment if you struggle with heavy weights. You can always increase or decrease the weight if you find certain moves too easy or too hard.

Q
DO I NEED TO GO TO A GYM?

A

While in the first four-week plan all you needed was a bit of time, space and motivation, to complete this advanced four-week plan you do need extra kit – namely a pair of dumbbells. If you have a set at home then great – you can do these workouts just like you did the first plan. If you don't, then you can buy a pair, or set, quite cheaply online. Alternatively, if you are a member of a gym, you can do you workouts there. Just find some space on the gym floor or in a studio, get the dumbbells you need, and set up your stopwatch!

Q
DO I CHANGE HOW AND WHAT I EAT?

A

If you followed our guide to eating for a better body, which began on p18, you'll know how easy it is to eat for better health. And the good news is that the leaner you are, the better able your body is to handle eating carbohydrates without storing the excess energy as fat. Therefore, when embarking on this advanced plan, you may want to eat a few more carbs on training days to give your body the energy it needs to train harder. You might also want to eat a bit more high-quality protein so your muscles can be repaired quickly.

Q
WHAT ELSE DO I NEED TO KNOW?

A

Each week of workouts is clearly explained before you begin, but follows a very similar structure to the initial plan, with three sessions per week of eight moves each, with a set time for work and a set time for rest for each exercise. Stick to the plan as closely as possible and see how far you can push yourself! Once you've completed this advanced plan you can simply repeat it again from the start, but using slightly heavier dumbbells to keep your muscles working hard so your body keeps burning fat and getting leaner!

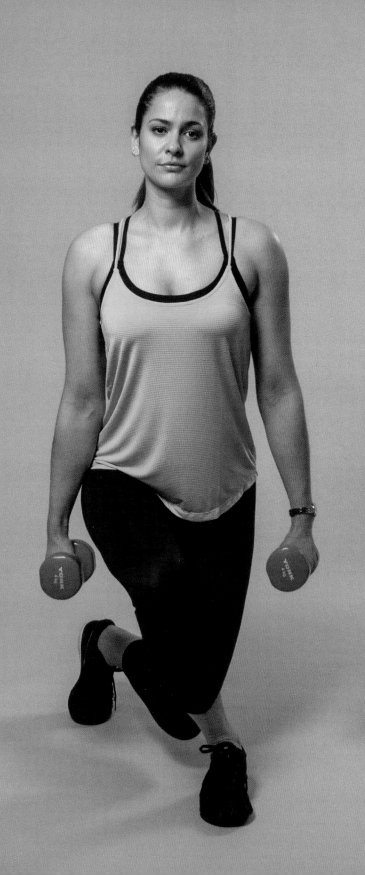

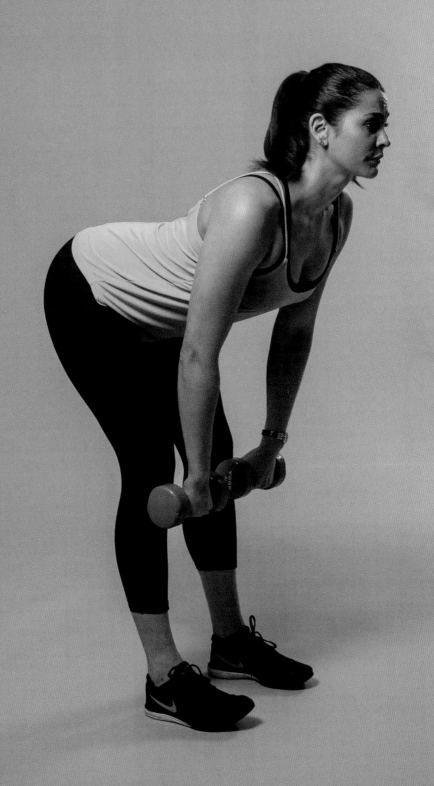

Are you ready for amazing results?

You're now ready to start the advanced version of the Four-Week Bikini Plan, and if you enjoyed the first month then you're in for a treat over the next 12 sessions! Yes, the workouts are harder and more challenging than in the first plan, but that means that if you apply yourself and give it all you've got you're going to make even more remarkable changes to your body - and feel better than ever!

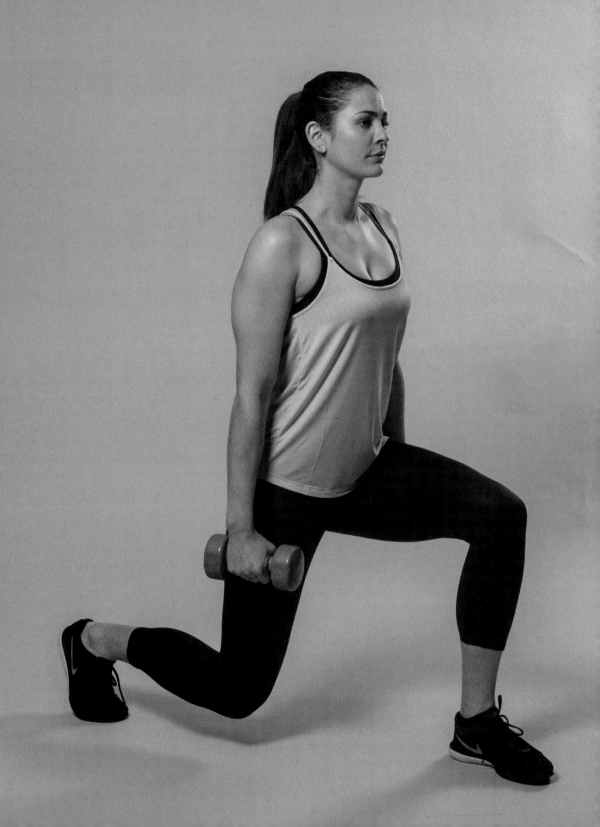

Weeks 1 + 2

Leave a day between each session in this, and every, week

For the first two weeks of this advanced four-week plan there are three total-body workouts, each comprising eight dumbbell or bodyweight moves. In week one you'll do four rounds of the circuit, but in week two you'll do an extra round, so five in total, to burn more body fat and further tone your muscles. Do the exercises in order, sticking to the work and rest periods detailed by each move's name. Let's go!

1 Dumbbell squat

TIME 30sec **REST** 30sec

DO 4 CIRCUITS IN WEEK 1 AND 5 IN WEEK 2

Stand tall holding a dumbbell in each hand by your sides then squat down, keeping your chest up and abs braced, until your hip crease is below the level of your knees. Drive back up through your heels.

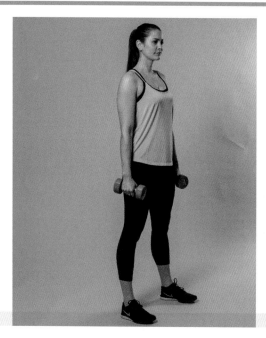
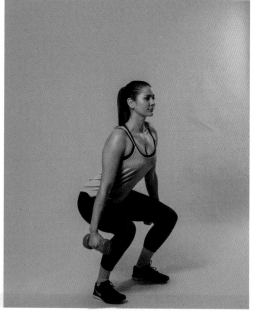

2 Dumbbell shoulder press

TIME 30sec **REST** 30sec

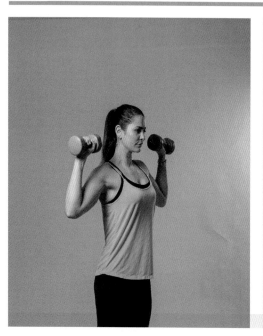
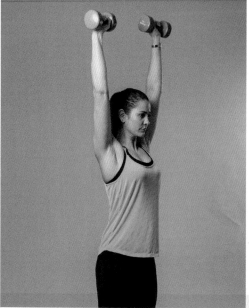

With your feet shoulder-width apart, hold a dumbbell in each hand at shoulder height. Keep your chest upright and your core muscles braced. Press the weights directly upwards, keeping your core braced, until your arms are extended overhead. Lower and repeat.

3 Dumbbell side lunge

TIME 30sec **REST** 30sec

Stand tall holding a dumbbell in each hand then take a big step sideways and bend your leading leg until your knee is at a right angle. Push off your leading foot to straighten your leg and return to the start position, then lunge to the other side leading with your other leg. Alternate sides with each rep.

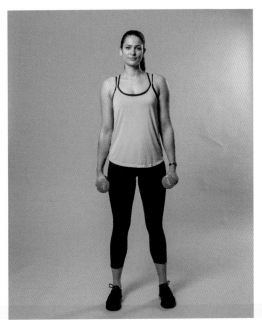
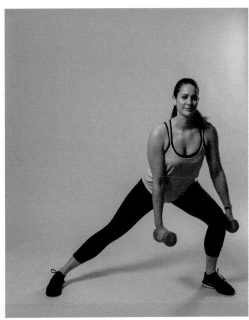

4 Dumbbell bent-over row

TIME 30sec **REST** 30sec

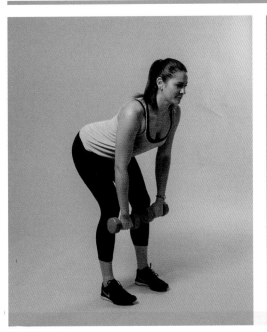
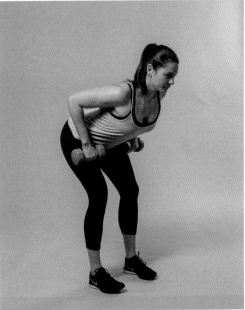

Stand with your core braced, your back straight and your shoulder blades retracted, holding a set of dumbbells, then bend your knees slightly and lean forwards from the hips. Pull the dumbbells up to just below stomach level. Pause, then lower under control.

5 **Dumbbell RDL**

TIME 30sec **REST** 30sec

Stand tall with your feet shoulder-width apart, holding a dumbbell in each hand. Keeping your legs straight, lean forward from the hips, not the waist, and lower the weights down the front of your legs until you feel a good stretch in your hamstrings. Reverse the move to the start and push your hips forward.

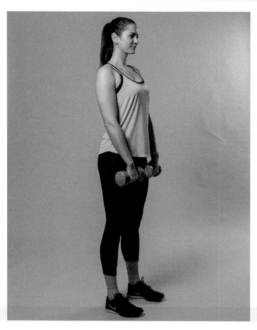
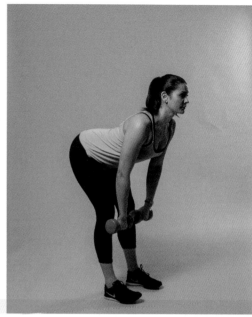

6 **Dumbbell biceps curl**

TIME 30sec **REST** 30sec

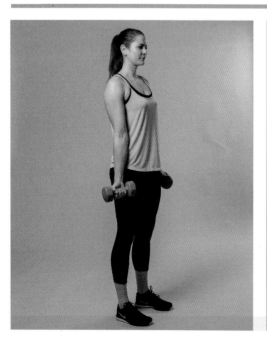
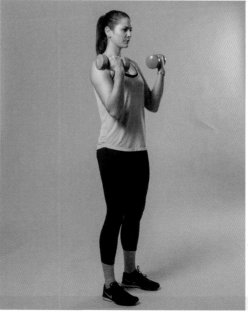

Stand tall holding a pair of dumbbells with palms facing forwards and hands just outside your hips. Keeping your elbows tucked in to your sides, curl the dumbbells up towards your chest, stopping just before your forearms reach vertical. Lower under control to return to the start position.

7 Dumbbell crunch

TIME 30sec **REST** 30sec

Lie flat on your back with knees bent and a dumbbell held at chest level. Contract your abs to lift your shoulders off the floor and curl your chest towards your knees. Pause at the top of the move and squeeze your abs, then lower slowly to the start.

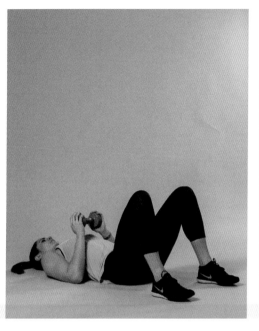 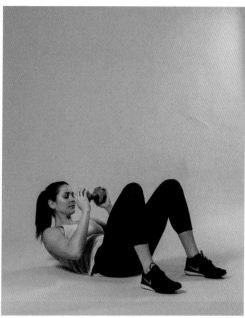

8 Dumbbell tall plank

TIME 30sec **REST** 2min

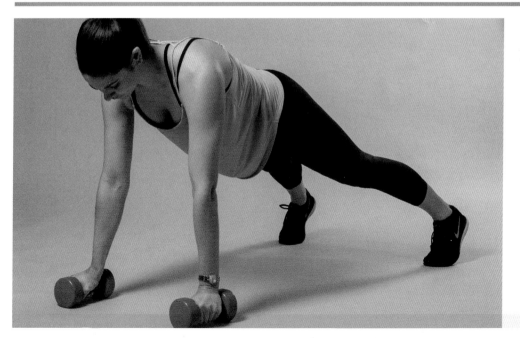

Get into position with your hands holding dumbbells with your wrists underneath your shoulders and your body in a straight line. Keep your abs and glutes (bum muscles) engaged to hold this position without letting your hips sag. Keep your breathing controlled and relaxed.

1 Goblet squat

TIME 40sec **REST** 20sec

DO 4 CIRCUITS IN WEEK 1 AND 5 IN WEEK 2

Hold a dumbbell or pair of dumbbells at chest height with both hands – like a goblet – then squat down until your elbows brush the insides of your knees. Keep your weight on your heels as you stand up.

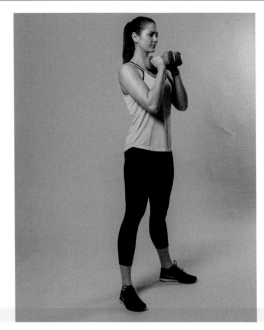
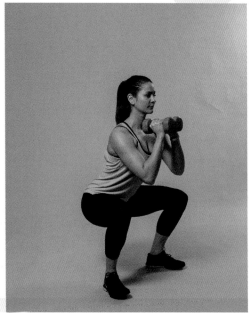

2 Dumbbell hammer press

TIME 40sec **REST** 20sec

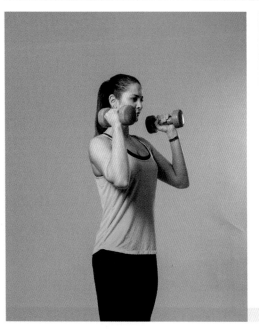
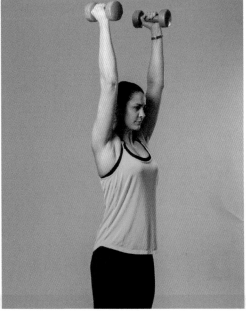

With your feet shoulder–width apart, hold a dumbbell in each hand at shoulder height with palms facing one another. Keep your chest upright and your core muscles braced. Press the weights directly upwards, keeping your core braced, until your arms are extended overhead. Lower and repeat.

3 Dumbbell curtsy squat

TIME 40sec **REST** 20sec

Stand tall with your chest up, holding a dumbbell in each hand by your sides. Keeping your chest up place one foot behind the other, then bend both knees to lunge down. Push off your rear foot to return to the start position, then repeat, leading with your other leg. Alternate legs with each rep.

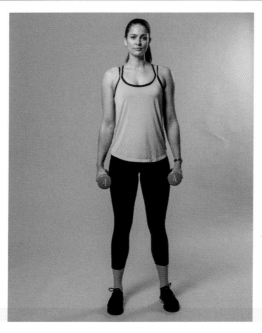
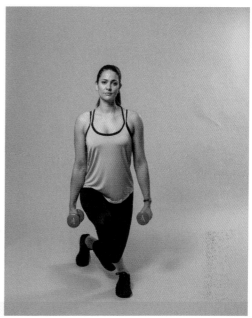

4 Dumbbell renegade row

TIME 40sec **REST** 20sec

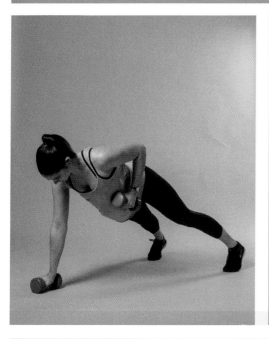
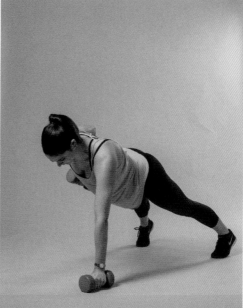

Start in a press-up position holding the handles of a pair of dumbbells. Row one dumbbell upwards and then back down, and then do the same with the other arm. Try to stay parallel to the floor and don't twist your hips as you row each arm up.

5 Dumbbell glute bridge

TIME 40sec **REST** 20sec

Lie flat on your back supporting a dumbbell in both hands on your hips. Tense your abs and glutes, then raise your hips until they're in line with your shoulders. Hold for a second in the top position, then lower.

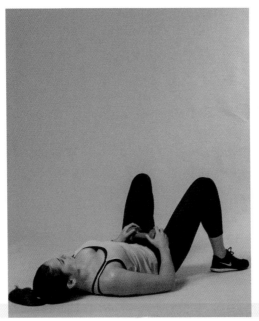
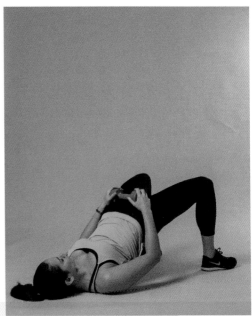

6 Dumbbell triceps extension

TIME 40sec **REST** 20sec

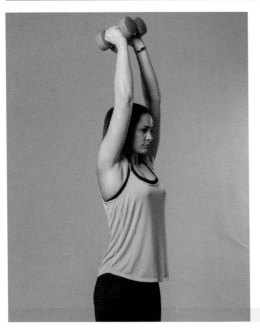
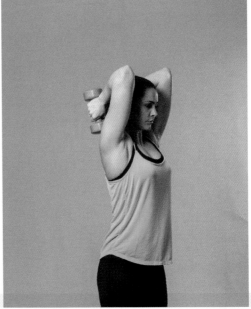

Stand tall, holding a dumbbell directly overhead in each hand. Keeping your chest up and abs engaged, lower the dumbbells down behind the back of your head by bending your elbows. Keep your elbows pointing directly up and keep your upper arms as still as possible.

7 Dumbbell leg raise

TIME 40sec **REST** 20sec

Lie on your back with your legs straight gripping a dumbbell between your feet. Engage your abs, then raise your feet off the floor. Keeping your legs straight, raise your feet as high as you can, then lower them back down.

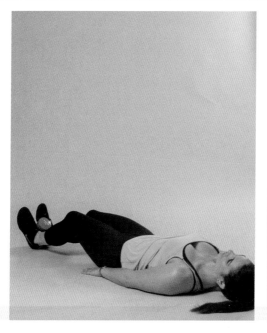
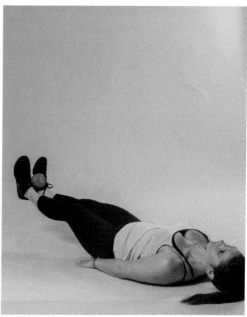

8 Dumbbell side plank star

TIME 40sec **REST** 2min

Lie on your side, supporting your upper body on your left forearm and holding a dumbbell in your right hand. Engage your abs, then raise your hips so that your body forms a straight line and raise your hand straight up. Halfway through the time switch sides.

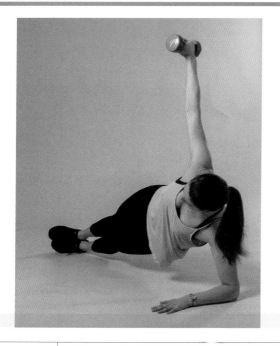

1 Dumbbell front squat

TIME 30sec **REST** 30sec

DO 4 CIRCUITS IN WEEK 1 AND 5 IN WEEK 2

Stand tall holding a dumbbell in each hand at shoulder height then squat down, keeping your chest up and abs braced, until your hip crease is below the level of your knees. Drive back up through your heels.

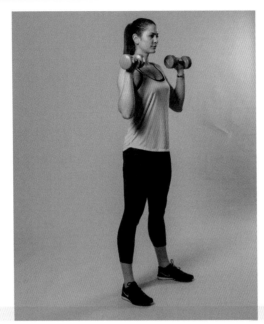 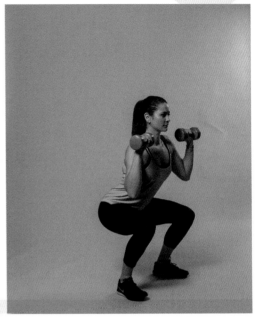

2 Dumbbell lateral raise

TIME 30sec **REST** 30sec

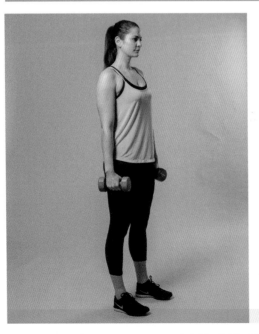 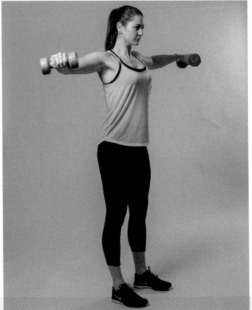

Stand tall with your abs braced and feet close together, holding a light dumbbell in each hand by your sides with your palms facing one another. Keeping a slight bend in your elbows, raise the weights out to the sides making sure you use your muscles and not momentum. Stop just below shoulder height, then lower.

3 Dumbbell lunge

TIME 30sec **REST** 30sec

Holding a dumbbell in each hand, take a big step forwards and lower your body until both knees are bent at right angles. Push off your front foot to reverse the movement back to the start, then repeat leading with your other leg. Alternate leading legs with each rep.

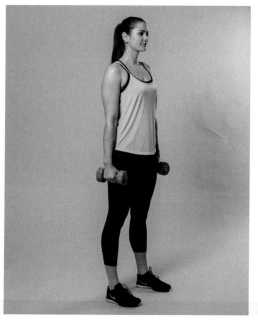
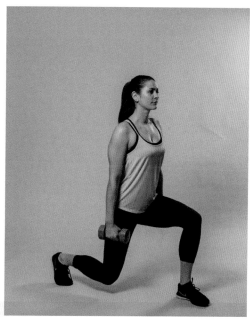

4 Underhand bent-over row

TIME 30sec **REST** 30sec

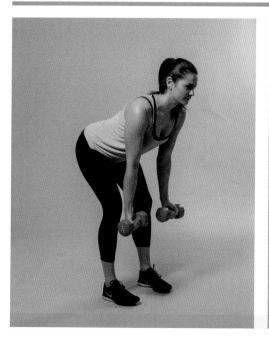
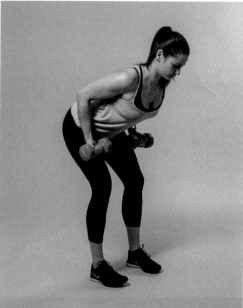

Stand with your core braced, your back straight and your shoulder blades retracted, holding a set of dumbbells with an underhand grip. Bend your knees slightly and lean forwards from the hips. Pull the dumbbells up to just below chest level. Pause, then lower under control.

5 Dumbbell RDL

TIME 30sec **REST** 30sec

Stand tall with your feet shoulder–width apart, holding a dumbbell in each hand. Keeping your legs straight, lean forward from the hips, not the waist, and lower the weights down the front of your legs until you feel a good stretch in your hamstrings. Reverse the move to the start and push your hips forward.

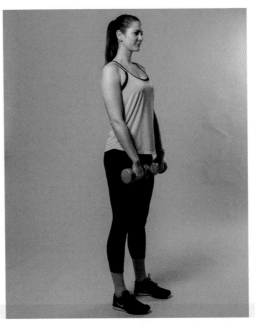
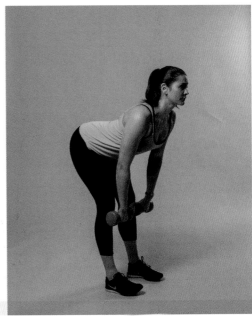

6 Dumbbell hammer curl

TIME 30sec **REST** 30sec

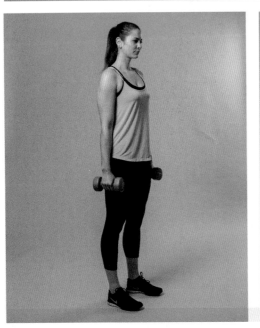
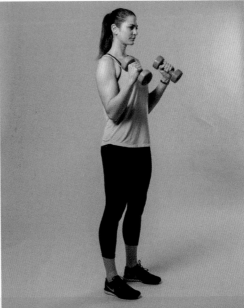

Stand tall with your shoulders back and feet close together, holding a pair of dumbbells with your palms facing your sides. Keeping your elbows tucked in to your sides, curl the dumbbells up to your chest. Lower under control to return to the start position.

7 **Dumbbell crunch reach**

TIME 30sec **REST** 30sec

Lie flat on your back with your knees bent and a dumbbell held above your chest with arms straight. Crunch upward, pausing at the top of the movement, then lower back to the start.

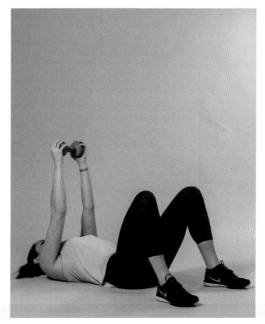
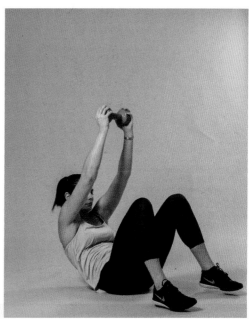

8 **Dumbbell leg lower hold**

TIME 30sec **REST** 2in

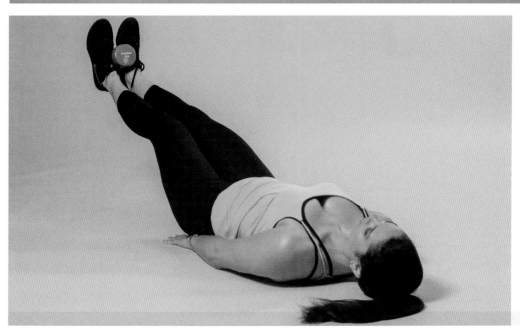

Lie flat on your back with your legs straight and a dumbbell gripped between your feet. Engage your abs, then raise your feet off the floor. Keeping your legs straight, raise your feet as high as you can. Keep your abs fully engaged to hold this position, keeping your breathing controlled.

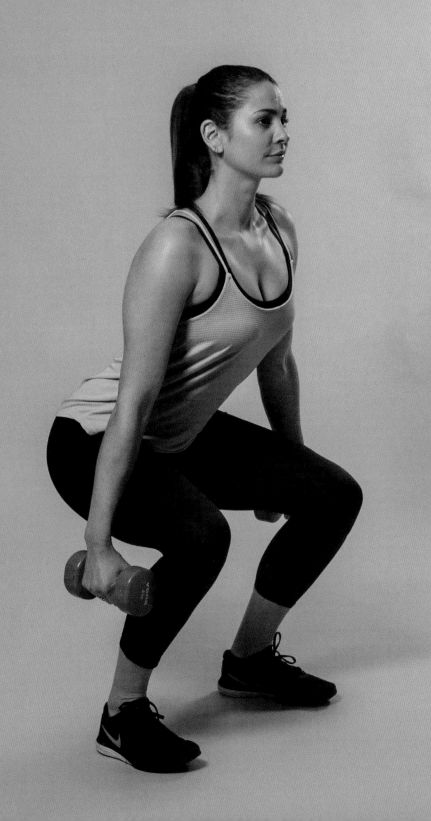

Weeks 3 + 4

Leave a day between each session in this, and every, week

It's the final fortnight of the advanced plan, so we've changed up all of the exercises - using a variety of more complex dumbbell and bodyweight moves - to make each session that little bit harder so you finish this training plan strong! In week three do four rounds of each circuit, then in week four do an extra round, so a total of five, to torch that last bit of body fat and add the final touches to your brand-new body!

1 Dumbbell floor press

TIME 30sec **REST** 30sec

DO 4 CIRCUITS IN WEEK 3 AND 5 IN WEEK 4

Lie flat on the floor with your knees bent holding a dumbbell in each hand with straight arms. Bend your elbows to lower the weights down towards your chest then press them back up powerfully.

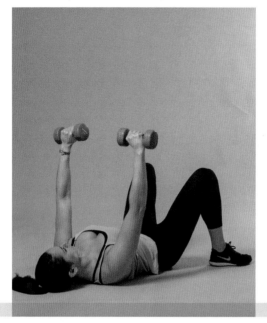
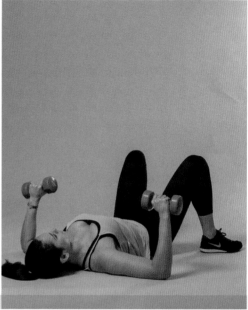

2 Dumbbell bent-over row

TIME 30sec **REST** 30sec

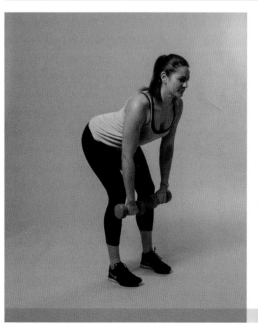
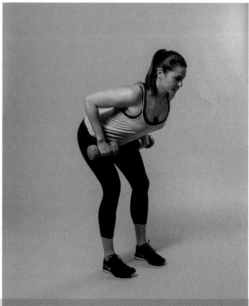

Stand with your core braced, your back straight and your shoulder blades retracted, holding a set of dumbbells, then bend your knees slightly and lean forwards from the hips. Row the dumbbells up to just below stomach level. Pause, then lower under control.

3 Dumbbell bent-over flye

TIME 30sec **REST** 30sec

Leaning forwards at the hips with a weight in each hand, keep your back flat and bring the weights upwards as if you were spreading your wings, aiming to bring your shoulder blades together at the top of the move.

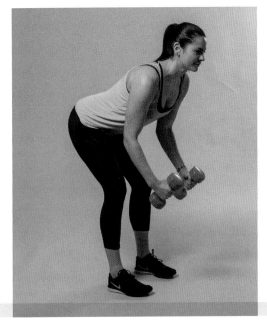
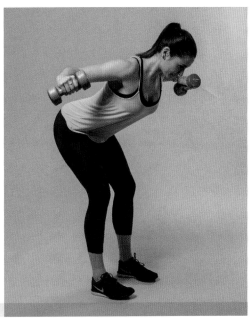

4 Dumbbell press-up

TIME 30sec **REST** 30sec

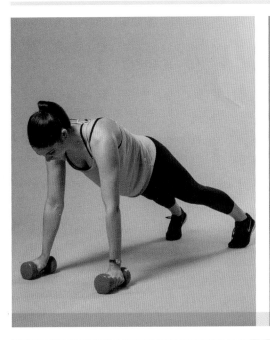
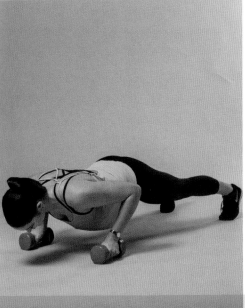

Start in a press-up position gripping the handles of a pair of dumbbells. Bend your elbows to lower your chest down towards the ground, then press back up powerfully to return to the start. Try to keep your body parallel to the floor and don't twist your hips as you press down and up.

5 Dumbbell renegade row

TIME 30sec **REST** 30sec

Start in a press-up position holding the handles of a pair of dumbbells. Row one dumbbell upwards and then back down, and then do the same with the other arm. Try to stay parallel to the floor and don't twist your hips as you row each arm up.

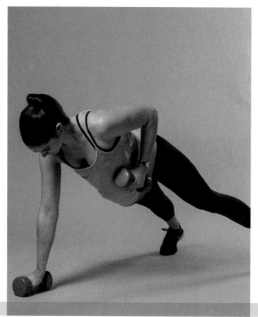
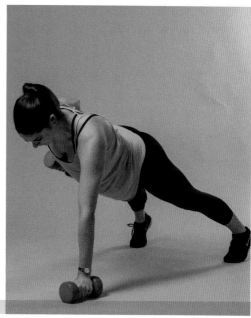

6 Crunch

TIME 30sec **REST** 30sec

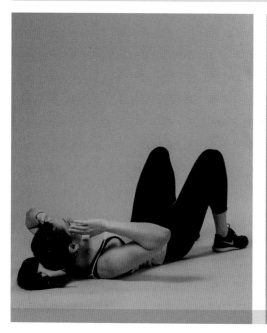
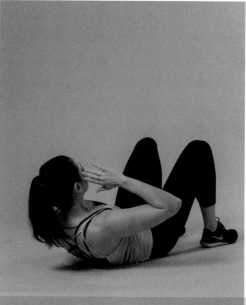

Lie flat on your back with your knees bent and feet flat on the floor, and bend your arms so your fingers touch your temples. Engage your abs, then raise your torso off the floor without tensing your neck. Keep that tension on your abs as you slowly lower your torso back to the floor.

7 Reverse crunch

TIME 30sec **REST** 30sec

Lie flat on your back with your arms flat on the floor and knees bent. Use your lower abs to draw your knees in towards your chest, then raise your hips up off the ground, then lower back to the start, keeping your abs fully engaged throughout.

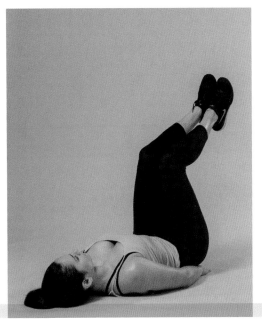
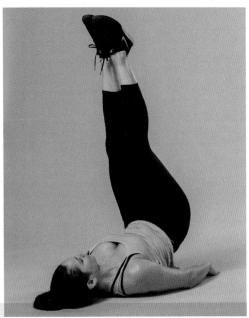
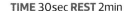

8 Plank

TIME 30sec **REST** 2min

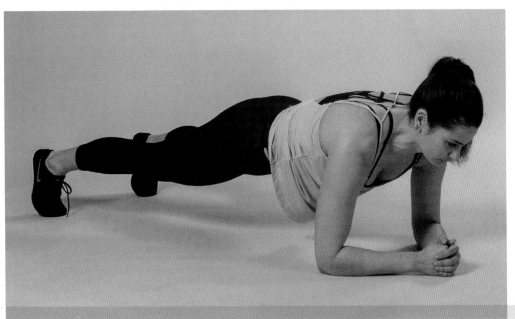

Get into position, supporting yourself on your forearms with your elbows underneath your shoulders. Engage your abs, then raise your hips so that your body forms a straight line from head to heels. Hold this position by keeping your abs and glutes engaged to prevent your hips from sagging.

1 Dumbbell squat

TIME 40sec **REST** 20sec

DO 4 CIRCUITS IN WEEK 3 AND 5 IN WEEK 4

Stand tall holding a dumbbell in each hand by your sides then squat down, keeping your chest up and abs braced, until your hip crease is below the level of your knees. Drive back up through your heels.

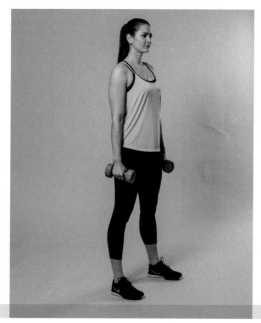
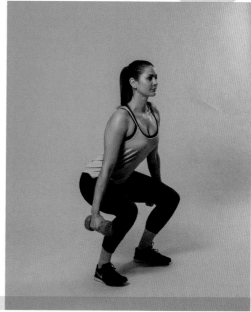

2 Dumbbell split squat - left

TIME 40sec **REST** 20sec

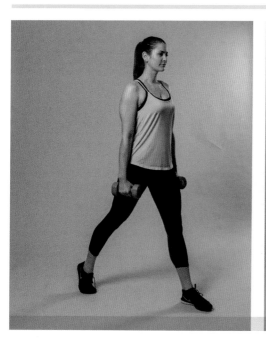
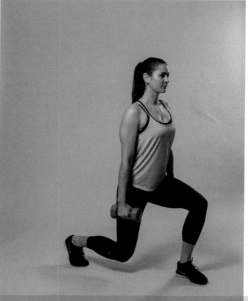

Start in a split stance, with your left foot in front of the other, holding a dumbbell in each hand. Bend both legs until your right knee almost touches the floor. Straighten both legs to return to the start, then go straight into the next rep.

3 Dumbbell split squat - right

TIME 40sec **REST** 20sec

Start in a split stance, with your right foot in front of the other, holding a dumbbell in each hand. Bend both legs until your left knee almost touches the floor. Straighten both legs to return to the start, then go straight into the next rep.

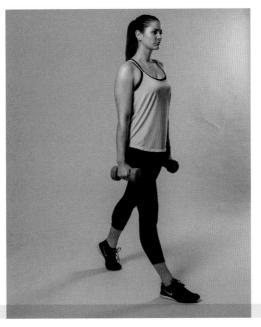
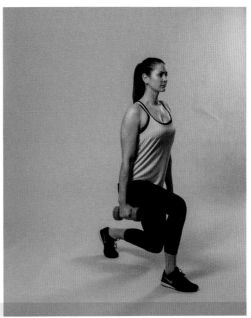

4 Dumbbell RDL

TIME 40sec **REST** 20sec

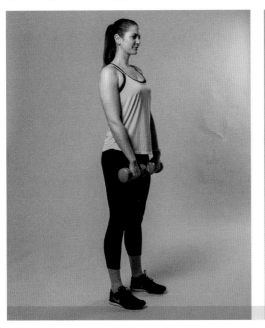
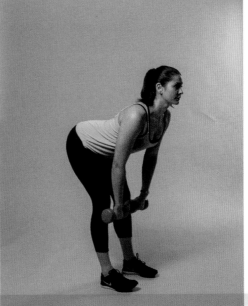

Stand tall with feet shoulder-width apart, holding a dumbbell in each hand. Keeping your legs straight, lean forward from the hips, not the waist, and lower the weights down the front of your legs until you feel a good stretch in your hamstrings. Reverse the move to the start and push your hips forward.

5 Dumbbell glute bridge

TIME 40sec **REST** 20sec

Lie flat on your back supporting a dumbbell in both hands on your hips. Tense your abs and glutes, then raise your hips until they're in line with your shoulders. Hold for a second in the top position, then lower.

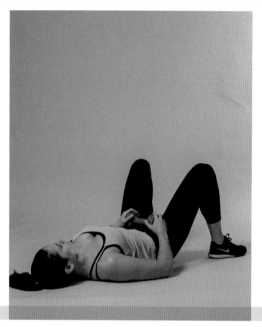
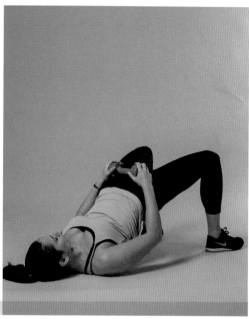

6 Mountain climbers

TIME 40sec **REST** 20sec

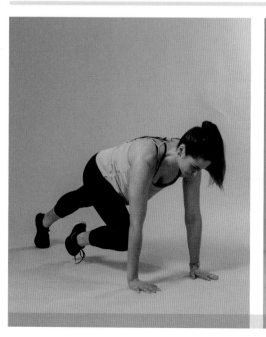
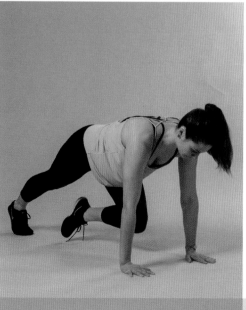

Get on all fours with your arms and legs straight. Without letting your hips sag, draw one knee up and bring it towards the elbow on the same side. Straighten that leg, then repeat, bringing your other knee towards your elbow. Keep your abs engaged throughout and keep the reps fast.

7 Dumbbell Russian twist

TIME 40sec **REST** 20sec

Sit on the floor with your knees bent and feet slightly raised, holding a dumbbell in front of you. Twist to one side, pause, and then twist to the other.

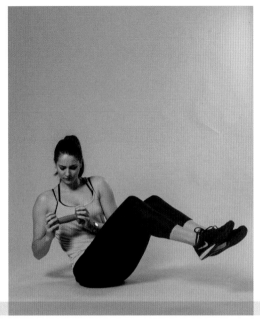
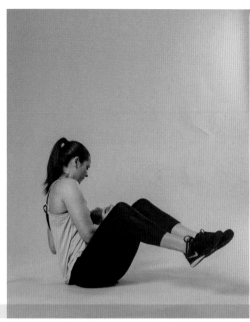

8 Dumbbell side plank star

TIME 40sec **REST** 2min

Lie on your side, supporting your upper body on your left forearm and holding a dumbbell in your right hand. Engage your abs, then raise your hips so that your body forms a straight line and raise your hand straight up. Halfway through the time switch sides.

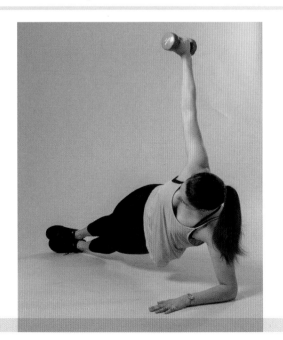

1 Dumbbell shoulder press

TIME 30sec **REST** 30sec

DO 4 CIRCUITS IN WEEK 3 AND 5 IN WEEK 4

With your feet shoulder-width apart, hold a dumbbell in each hand at shoulder height. Keep your chest upright and your core muscles braced. Press the weights directly upwards, keeping your core braced, until your arms are extended overhead. Lower and repeat.

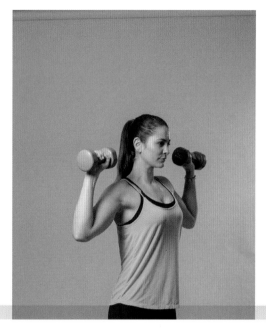
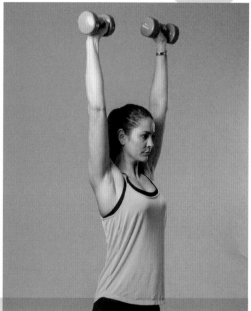

2 Dumbbell lateral raise

TIME 30sec **REST** 30sec

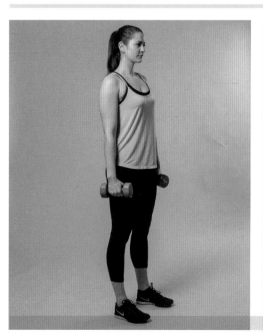
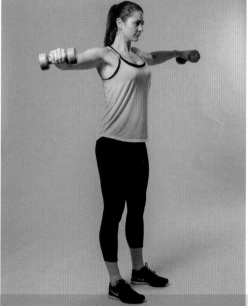

Stand tall with your abs braced holding a light dumbbell in each hand by your sides with your palms facing one another. Keeping a slight bend in your elbows, raise the weights out to the sides making sure you use your muscles and not momentum. Stop just below shoulder height, then lower.

3 Dumbbell triceps extension

TIME 30sec **REST** 30sec

Stand tall, holding a dumbbell directly overhead in each hand. Keeping your chest up and abs engaged, lower the dumbbells down behind the back of your head by bending your elbows. Keep your elbows pointing directly up and keep your upper arms as still as possible.

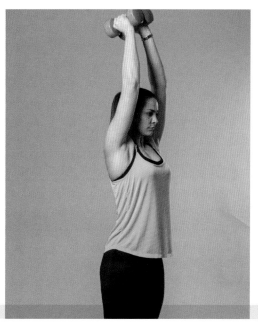
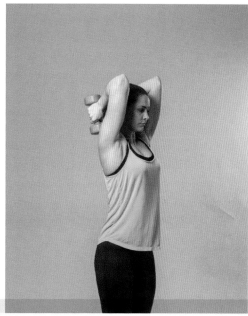

4 Dumbbell triceps kickback

TIME 30sec **REST** 30sec

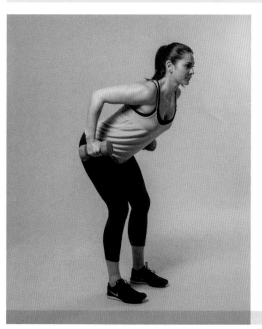
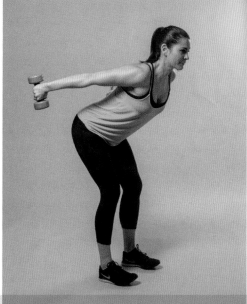

Stand tall holding a dumbbell in each hand with your elbows bent so the weights are at chest height. Lean forwards from the hips and, keeping your chest up, straighten both arms back and behind you. Bend your elbows to return the weights back in and repeat. Do one arm at a time if you need to make the move easier.

5 Dumbbell biceps curl

TIME 30sec REST 30sec

Stand tall holding a pair of dumbbells with palms facing forwards and hands just outside your hips. Keeping your elbows tucked in to your sides, curl the dumbbells up towards your chest, stopping just before your forearms reach vertical. Lower under control to return to the start position.

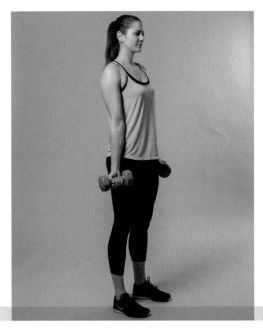
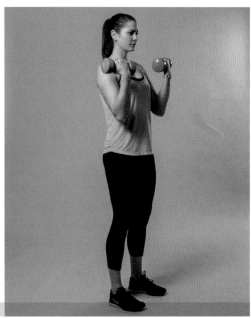

6 Dumbbell hammer curl

TIME 30sec REST 30sec

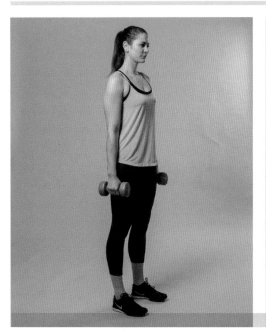
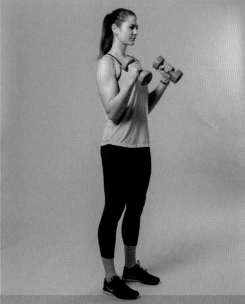

Stand tall holding a pair of dumbbells with your palms facing your sides. Keeping your elbows tucked in to your sides, curl the dumbbells up towards your chest, stopping just before your forearms reach vertical. Lower under control to return to the start position.

7 Dumbbell crunch reach

TIME 30sec **REST** 30sec

Lie flat on your back with your knees bent and a dumbbell held above your chest with arms straight. Crunch upward, pausing at the top of the movement, then lower back to the start.

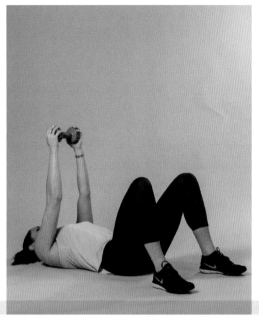
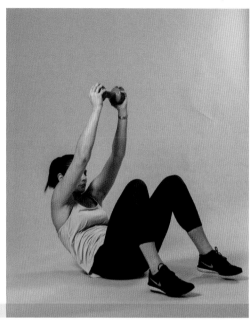

8 Dumbbell jackknife

TIME 30sec **REST** 2min

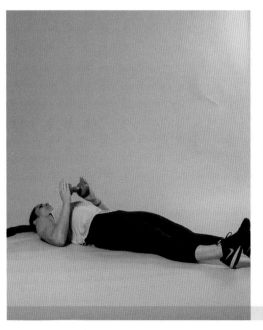
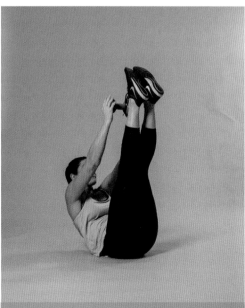

Lie flat on your back with your legs straight holding a dumbbell above your chest. Engage your abs. Raise your feet off the floor, and bring your arms forwards so the weight touches your legs. Try and reach as far up your leg as possible to work your abs harder.

OUR TOP 3 HEALTH PICKS

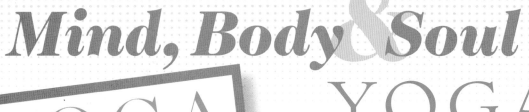

Mind, Body & Soul

YOGA
A beginner's guide

Until you've experienced it for yourself it's hard to really understand the difference regular yoga practice can make to your life. People speak of improved flexibility, increased strength, better balance and greater stamina, but the benefits go far beyond the physical. Along with better sleep, deeper relaxation, greater focus and increased feelings of calm, yoga can give you a sense of purpose and belonging that is hard to beat. This step-by-step guide leads you through the foundations of yoga, including postures, breathing technique and correct alignment, and offers an easy progression plan to take you from yoga newbie to practiced yogi.

Sneak peek of what's inside

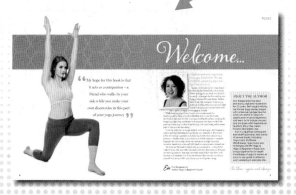

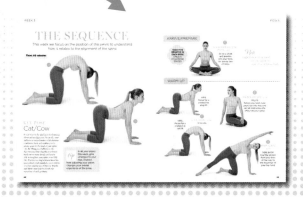